Stanley Zengeya
Geoffrey Meads

Four years since its introduction where is Choose and Book (C&B)

AF190945

Stanley Zengeya
Geoffrey Meads

Four years since its introduction where is Choose and Book (C&B)

What are the challenges facing frontline GPs and hospital consultants in its implementation

LAP LAMBERT Academic Publishing

Imprint

Any brand names and product names mentioned in this book are subject to trademark, brand or patent protection and are trademarks or registered trademarks of their respective holders. The use of brand names, product names, common names, trade names, product descriptions etc. even without a particular marking in this work is in no way to be construed to mean that such names may be regarded as unrestricted in respect of trademark and brand protection legislation and could thus be used by anyone.

Cover image: www.ingimage.com

Publisher:
LAP LAMBERT Academic Publishing
is a trademark of
Dodo Books Indian Ocean Ltd. and OmniScriptum S.R.L publishing group

120 High Road, East Finchley, London, N2 9ED, United Kingdom
Str. Armeneasca 28/1, office 1, Chisinau MD-2012, Republic of Moldova, Europe
Managing Directors: Ieva Konstantinova, Victoria Ursu
info@omniscriptum.com

Printed at: see last page
ISBN: 978-3-659-36317-7

Zugl. / Approved by: Warwick. University of Warwick, Dissertation September, 2010

PROFESSIONAL PROJECT

Title:

Four years since its introduction where is Choose and Book (C&B)?

What are the challenges facing frontline GPs and hospital consultants in its

implementation?

"This project report has been submitted to the University of Warwick in partial

fulfilment of the requirements for the award of the degree of MSc Health

Sciences –Management"

Student Identification Number: *0758410*

Word Count: *10869*

Month and Year of Submission: *September 2010*

1

Four years since its introduction where is Choose and Book (C&B)?

What are the challenges facing frontline GPs and hospital consultants in its implementation?

CONTENTS   PAGE

Tables & Illustrations

Abbreviations

BREC- Biomedical and Scientific Research Committee

C&B - Choose and Book

CAB- Choose and Book

DGH - District General Hospital

DH – Department of Health

DNA- "Did not attend" appointment

GP- General Practitioner

NHS - National Health Service

NPfIT- National Programme for Information Technology

Appendices

Appendix 1   -Audit Report for the local trust hospital (Tables & Histograms removed)

Acknowledgements

I thank my family for their sacrifice during the time I was studying for this master's degree without which I could not have achieved this task especially my wife Anna and my children. They were my source of strength to undertake this project.

I thank my supervisor Professor Geoffrey Meads for his tremendous support and guidance throughout this project. His focused approach and wealth of experience enabled me to complete this project.

I thank the Trust Data Analyst who worked tirelessly to provide all the data on referrals to the Outpatient Department

I thank Sharon Edwards and the trust audit department for help ng with data compilation and storage for trust-wide dissemination.

Declaration
I certify that this project is my own original work. It has not been published in any scientific journal before.

Abstract

Choose and Book is a central part of the UK Government patient choice agenda.

Aims & Objectives: This study was a service evaluation of the professional medical staff's use of the Choose and Book system at a local NHS trust.

Methods: Data of all referrals to the outpatient department was retrospectively extracted from January 2008 to December 2009. A simple questionnaire was designed using online survey software. This was disseminated electronically to all local general practitioners and hospital consultants to obtain data and feedback for analysis.

Results: At the end of study period 51% of all referral were through C&B. GPs vary considerably in the extent to which they actively support patient choice. Most patients were referred to a specialty not a named consultant. Some local GP practices were not using C&B at all. DNA rates were marginally better with C&B. Some hospital specialties received higher numbers of referrals through C&B compared to others

Questionnaire: Only 7% of respondents thought that C&B improved patient care. Short waiting time and easy access were considered by GPs to be most important factors for patients. 17.5% of respondents were using C&B for all their patients while 22.5% of respondents did not use C&B for any of their patients. C&B had many associated technical problems and was not user friendly. Only a quarter of respondents were satisfied with the use of C&B, with at least 50% expressing either dissatisfaction or extreme dissatisfaction. There was a lack of sufficient choice, either of hospitals or specialists on offer in the rural setting.

Conclusion: Medical professionals need to embrace the principle of "patient choice" as paramount and that it is here to stay. There is a need for a change in culture within the NHS for C&B to be implemented at a more rapid pace.

Chapter 1

Introduction:

Improving the quality of health care and services is a priority for the NHS, and for commissioners, managers, practitioners and service users. However, to improve we must first know what already exists. The primary way to do this is to measure what is being provided by evaluating current services.

"It is only through measuring what we do .... that teams can improve the quality of care for patients – by capturing data and harnessing technology, making information available to the whole team and taking collective responsibility for the results." (Department of Health, 2009, p27)

The importance of dissemination of any evaluation work cannot be over emphasised. It is only by sharing our learning that we can improve services.

There is a widely held view by healthcare professionals, especially hospital consultants, that the Choose and Book system does not seem to deliver the improvements in patient choice that it was intended to when it was first introduced (Oates 2007). At its inception Choose and Book had three separate elements of innovation combined. Through the NHS Improvement Plan, eligible patients were assured of a clinically appropriate choice from at least four hospitals or a suitable alternative provider when referred for a specialist outpatient opinion. The ultimate goal was for consumers to have 'free choice' and all referral to be made through C&B by 2008, but in 2010 this is not the case. Secondly patients would be allowed to book a mutually convenient appointment. Thirdly Choose and Book was also aimed at assisting clinicians and patients in making appropriate choices and booking convenient appointments.(NHS Direct website). GPs are now expected to help patients choose where they attend for a specialist appointment or further treatment, and this role looks set to expand (NHS website)

Background:

After a 2004 pilot study, the system was installed into nearly every GP practice during 2005 and went live across the country on 1 January 2006. It was introduced as part of NHS improvement plan (DH, 2004). It seeks to provide patients with a choice over the time, date and place of their first outpatient appointment with a specialist. Choose and Book was one of the DH's (NPfIT) vanguard initiatives. The NHS NPfIT is the largest of such systems in the world (Brenan, 2005). Its aim was to transform the old booking system by combining, for the first time, electronic booking with patient choice of their first hospital appointment. A significant criticism in the National Audit Office report was that procurement occurred before clinical engagement, perhaps because extensive consultation was thought to slow the process (Coiera, 2007). This has resulted in significant disquiet among some clinicians and the priorities of the program not fully matching those of the clinical community (Hendy et al, 2005).

Choose and Book is an international example of both the introduction of a large-scale medical informatics system and of a government policy to deliver patient choice. DH (2006) on its paper on patient choice, set out to offer patients choice at the point of referral. Rashid et al (2007) found that Choose and Book was still poorly perceived by doctors particularly with respect to technical problems and doctors' use of the system has been reported as being persistently low.

Choice policy has met with a mixed reaction from doctors, and while medical institutions such as the BMA and the Royal Colleges have accepted the principle, practising clinicians have often struggled with their own philosophical uncertainty and practical constraints. Those of a rather paternalistic consulting style have found it particularly difficult to accept that patients should be encouraged to assert their own view of where they might receive treatment. They doubt that patients can be sufficiently informed to make a 'better' choice than their expert doctor. Enthusiasts have seen choice as an important way to involve and empower patients and to put pressure on hospitals to be more responsive to patients' needs. There is still some support for the concept of electronic booking; however the patient choice element faces more resistance (Walford, 2006).

Wood (2006) described how Choose and Book appointment system had been imposed with detrimental effects. Furthermore, UK general practitioners have no contractual obligation to offer patients a choice of provider (Coombes 2006). Lewis (2006) in his letter to the BMJ argues that the current compensation for implementing C&B is meagre for GPs who must devote additional time and effort to assist staff to implement Choose and Book for their patients, although evidence of the clinical benefit for patients is lacking. The additional time per appointment that may ensue reduces their overall availability to see patients, thus jeopardising their facility to see everyone within 48 hours. He wonders whether this is really the way to maintain morale in general practice and support an already overstretched service.

A pertinent question with regards to C&B is whether patients want choice. Current policies suggest that choice empowers patients and drives up standards within the NHS (Coulter, 2003). The notion that the concept of consumerism can be applied to healthcare seems plausible given patient's desire for choice (Appleby 2005, DOH 2003). Despite this clinicians have often been dismissive of the general notion that patients want choice. Research in this field is inconclusive as to exactly what patients do want, but it leaves little doubt that the opportunity to make choice for oneself is highly valued. Additional research is needed on this topic to further investigate the use of electronic systems in the health service. Green et al (2007) in their study found that patients did not experience the degree of choice that Choose and Book was designed to deliver in terms of the timing, date and place of their first outpatient appointment. This study was performed soon after (in January 2006) the implementation of this system.

Bryant (2007) argues that while choice is a good thing, it is the quality of information given to the user which determines whether choice is a good thing or not. GPs play a key role in this process. This is why in this project GPs' views were sought on how C&B implementation could be improved. The language that is used should be simple for the patient to understand and emphasis should be placed on decisions and consequences rather than just offering a choice. Simply offering more choice may adversely affect the quality of decisions made (Schwartz, 2004).

Lakhani and Baker (2006) describe a vision for general practice where GPs might see themselves more as 'navigators' than 'gatekeepers' in the modern NHS. They emphasise a patient-centred approach where clinicians would be supported by highly developed strategic organisations collaborating with each other in a community network. C&B was supposed to revolutionise the old booking system, with patients for the first time being able to choose their initial hospital appointment and book it at their convenience. Coincidentally, the NHS would save money on 'Did Not Attends' (DNAs) and administration, while doctors would benefit from being able to track referrals and have more efficient referral information with none of the delays of paper correspondence.

Despite C&B's theoretical advantages published data shows conflicting results, Parmer et al (2009) in a large audit in an Audiology Medicine Clinic found that when compared to the traditional method of booking, C&B resulted in reduced number of DNAs. This audit suggests that when primary care agents book outpatient clinic appointments online it improves outpatient attendance. 'Choose and Book' patients had a significantly better rate of attendance than traditional appointment patients'. However, Modayil et al (2009) in a setting of an orthopaedic clinic found that the DNA rates with C&B were worse than those of traditional referrals. In a pilot study at their hospital they observed a significant difference of 18% (C&B) compared to 12% (paper referral) for non-attendance in clinics. Their conclusion was that C&B had failed to achieve its main goal of improving patients' satisfaction and attendance. Moreover, it creates an unnecessary economic burden on the health system and jeopardises the prioritisation process by removing clinicians from the process.

Bentley and Fletcher (2007) analysed the impact of C&B on the elderly who are major users of the NHS. They found some significant variations in use in different age groups which might negatively affect its implementation.

The British Medical Association (2007) said in a statement published at their annual conference, "the NHS's Choose and Book system is unfit for purpose and actually limits choice for patients". Doctors at the BMA's Annual General Meeting voted for an investigation into the impact Choose and Book on referrals. BMA members described the system as politically motivated and designed to help meet targets. One consultant told the conference that he rejects about half of C&B appointments because they do not match his skills or are for patients already being cared for by colleagues. But other attendees blamed the way Primary Care Trusts implement C&B for the problems, not the system itself.

Rabiei et al (2009) in their study found that although clinicians were positive about the benefits of the C&B service, they were concerned about the adverse impact of the electronic referral process on their jobs. They conclude that paying attention to the impact of the service on clinicians' jobs, at both ends of the process, could help to improve the referral process and the use of the system. Similarly Pothier et al (2006) found that

10

the majority of GPs were not in favour of Choose and Book. Many cited difficulties with time constraints and an inflexible system as factors that made Choose and Book unacceptable.

Since April 2008, the scheme has been further expanded with the Free Choice policy under which most patients should be able to choose from any secondary care provider (NHS or independent sector) across England (DH, 2008). From April 2009, it has become a legal right for patients to choose any hospital which meets NHS standards where they can receive medical care including private hospitals. We carried out a service evaluation of C&B implementation at a large local NHS trust to explore the views of GPs and hospital consultants on possible reasons for the delay in its full implementation.

Chapter 2

AIM AND OBJECTIVES

Aim:

This study was aimed at evaluating the medical professional response to the Choose and Book system at a local NHS trust.

Objectives:

This project was designed to evaluate the use of Choose and Book as a referral system within the NHS using a local trust as an example.

Our objectives were to:

1. Establish the current referral pattern to a large DGH
2. Establish what percentage of referrals were made through C&B
3. Identify the DNA rates for C&B patients compared to paper copy referrals
4. Identify the views of local healthcare providers (GPs and consultants) on the use of Choose and Book system
5. Explore what were the contributing factors to the slow pace of C&B implementation
6. Explore some management tools that could be used to improve C&B implementation.
7. Provide recommendations to improve C&B implementation for inclusion in PCT terms of commissioning.

Definitions

Choose and Book is a service that allows the patient to choose their hospital or clinic for their first appointment to see a specialist. (NHS Direct website)

When a GP and a patient agree that a specialist appointment is required Choose and Book shows the GP which hospitals or clinics are available for treatment. The GP discusses with the patient what clinically appropriate options are available for their treatment. Patients make a choice according to what matters most to them, whether it's location, waiting times, reputation, clin cal performance, visiting policies, parking facilities or other patients' comments.

Service evaluation is defined as:

"A set of procedures to judge a services merit by providing a systematic assessment of its aims, objectives, activities, outputs, outcomes and costs". (NHS Executive, 1997).

Service evaluation is a way to define or measure current practice within the NHS. This evaluation should have a purpose: why we are measuring and what information we want to get out of the process before selecting a tool. Choose and Book has now been in use for at least four years and hence relevant evaluation to assess its use is necessary to benefit those who use this particular service. The participants are those who use the service or deliver it. In this evaluation we assessed the service from the point of view of the GPs who deliver C&B and hospital consultants who receive these referrals.

The results of this evaluation were used to produce some internal recommendations for improvements that are not intended to be generalised beyond the setting in which the evaluation took place. The service evaluation was designed to answer the question: what standard was this service achieving?

Clinical audit:

This project used primarily clinical audit tools as defined by NICE (2002). Clinical audit is about improving services. One definition that is used is:

"Clinical audit is a quality improvement process that seeks to improve patient care and outcomes through systematic review of care against explicit criteria and the implementation of change." (NICE, 2002, Principles for Best Practice in Clinical Audit, p.1)

Clinical audit is a continuous process and re-audit aims to measure care against criteria and assess the impact of the implementation of change. Audit asks the following questions:

- Is what is happening what should be happening?
- Are we doing what the evidence says we should be doing?
- Does practice meet the standards that have been set?
- Does practice follow published guidelines?
- Is knowledge or best evidence being applied in practice?

Clinical audit is designed to answer the question: Does this service reach a predetermined standard? The results of clinical audit help enforce good clinical practice and produce internal recommendations for any necessary improvements.

Literature Search:

Textbooks from the Warwick Library were used as an information resource. Electronic literature search of various business databases was made including Emerald, Business Premier and IngentaConnect, Illunmina, and EBSCO. Medline and Google Scholar were specifically searched for medical related literature. Searches were then made within specific management journals such as Managing Service Quality and the Harvard Business Review. The websites of Department of Health Website, NHS Direct, the NHS Institute for Innovation and Improvement were searched for relevant articles.

Search terms used included; Choose & Book, patient choice, healthcare 'user or consumer' hospital Information systems, information technology, quality improvement, patient referral systems, quality improvement, management tools, change management and 'culture of organisations'. Search period was from 1985 onwards.

Process of Choose and Book at the GP surgery and at the local hospital (Figures 1 & 2):

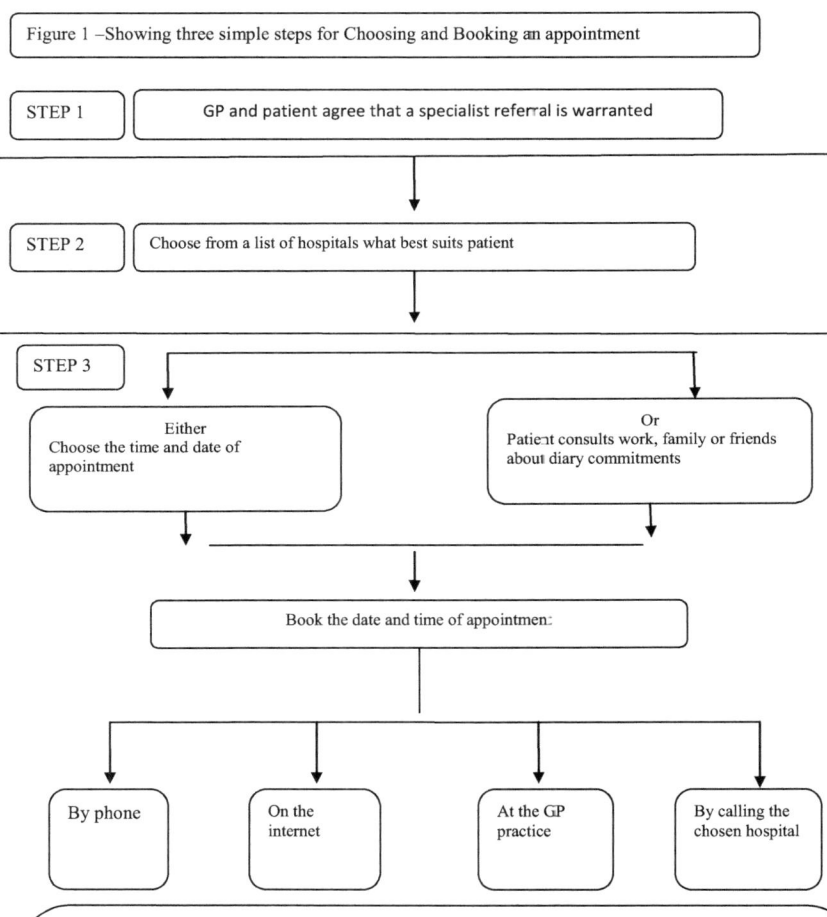

Figure 1 –Showing three simple steps for Choosing and Booking an appointment

STEP 1 — GP and patient agree that a specialist referral is warranted

STEP 2 — Choose from a list of hospitals what best suits patient

STEP 3

Either
Choose the time and date of appointment

Or
Patient consults work, family or friends about diary commitments

Book the date and time of appointment

By phone

On the internet

At the GP practice

By calling the chosen hospital

Referring clinician creates an Appointment Request by selecting a shortlist suited to the patient's clinical needs and preferences from a Directory of Services. Patients then book from a list of available slots in one of three ways:

- As part of or following the consultation, the GP or one of the practice staff uses the Choose and Book system to make an appointment while the patient is in the surgery.

- Patient accesses Choose and Book through the Web-based Patient Portal within NHS Healthspace and books for themselves, using their UBRN; or

- Patient calls the Booking Management Service quoting a unique booking reference number (UBRN)

Literature search:

Figure 2 showing the process of Choose and Book at the local trust hospital:

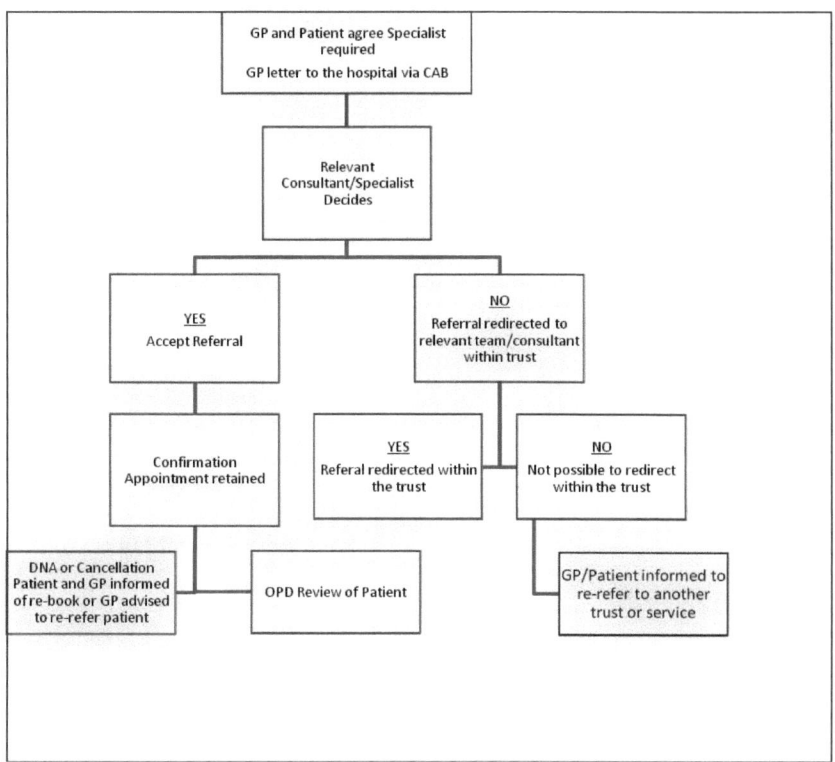

Chapter 3

Methods:

The Ethics Committee at the local hospital was contacted about this service evaluation exercise but advised that formal ethical approval was not required as there was no direct patient contact and referred this evaluation to the local audit department which agreed to lend its fill support to this and helped to set it up and assist with the data storage and dissemination. BREC approval was obtained through the University of Warwick Research Department. Data of all referrals to a large local NHS trust seen in the outpatient department (OPD) was retrospectively extracted from a two year period between January 2008 and December, 2009. This data was provided by the trust Choose and Book manager who collects all C&B data and compiles quarterly reports. Patients were grouped into whether they were referred using Choose and Book or the traditional "paper" referral system. Data was analysed for whether the referrals were "appropriate" or "inappropriate". Inappropriate referrals were those that required reallocation of specialists or clinics as deemed necessary by the hospital. The data was anonymised for patients, GPs or hospital consultants. No patient identifying data was collected.

The data was analysed to determine trends in referral patterns; proportions of patients within each group who did not attend (DNA); whether those referred using C&B were re-allocated to other services and whether any existing government targets were being met. The data was divided into quarterly intervals and then summed up into annual totals to show trends during the study period.

The data was further subdivided according to specialties and analysed to assess in which specialties C&B implementation was higher compared to those with lower rates of C&B referrals.

The second part of this project explored the views of GPs and hospital consultants on the possible reasons why C&B implementation was slower than anticipated and how this could be improved. This was done using a questionnaire. The questionnaire comprised ten stem questions with multiple options in each, exploring different themes involved in understanding the process of implementing C&B. Participants were expected to complete all relevant questions depending on whether they were GPs or hospital consultants. Given the timescales and the general acceptance of Choose and Book as appropriate for service evaluation, no pilot study was necessary.

Questionnaire

All local eligible GPs (approximately 100) and all hospital consultants (150), located within the boundaries of a single Borough who may or may not have used C&B were asked to complete a survey stating their views and opinions on the implementation of CAB using a questionnaire (See Appendix 1). These healthcare professionals were contacted using available emailing lists for both Consultants and GPs. To maximise the number of responses all local GPs and all consultants were invited to participate. We included all GPs and consultants including those who may not have used C&B to obtain as wide range of views as possible.

The questionnaire was electronically accessible on line using the Monkey Surveys online services. This is a secure service which is now widely used by the medical fraternity to carry out surveys. An email was sent out to local GPs and hospital consultants who were all available from local e-mail address list from the hospital intranet and the local GP network inviting them to complete the questionnaire using an online link. (See Appendix 1)

Only one response per e-mail address was allowed. GPs and hospital consultants were contacted using only their official registered NHS e-mail account ending with .nhs.uk. or nhs.net. The local hospital trust holds e-mail addresses of all hospital consultants which is secure. GP addresses were obtained from the local NHS GP network links. Responses were anonymous. Respondents are not aware of other people's responses and did not have access to the data.

Results of the survey were stored on a secure website (Monkey surveys) which was password protected and could not be accessed except by the investigator. Data was downloaded and analysed jointly with the audit department. After data gathering and analysis was complete the survey was deleted from the website. Data was analysed using quantitative methods but the free text comments from the questionnaire were analysed using grounded theory principles of coding and theme abstraction (Miles, 1979), rather than strict adherence to the theory of Glaser and Strauss (1967).

Chapter 4

Results:

All data of referrals to a local NHS trust is compiled in tables 1-6. The data was supplied in financial year format, (which starts in April) instead of the normal calendar year. The data is provided subdivided into quarterly intervals making it easier to observe any changes in the referral patterns.

There were a total of 129 556 (Table 1) referrals to the local hospital of which 52,883 (40.82%) were through C&B and 76,673 (59.18%) were through paper referrals (Table 6). There was a significant rise in the number of referrals using C&B by the end of the audit period. At the start of the audit period only 4,398 (29.8%) were referred using C&B versus 10,351(70.2%) by paper referral. By the end of the period in the third quarter of financial year 2009/10 there were 7,340 (51.6%) C&B referrals compared to 6,875 (48.4%) paper referrals (See Table 1) i.e. more than half of the referrals were made using C&B.

Table 2 shows the "did not attend" (DNA) rates of the two groups. The DNA rate for C&B referrals at the start of the audit was 4.4% compared to 6.0% for the paper referred patients. This trend continued throughout the whole audit period reaching 8.2% for C&B compared to 9.6% for paper referrals. The number of DNAs for both groups gradually increased during the study period (Table 2)

Patients referred using C&B showed much lower cancellation rates for their appointments compared to those patients referred using paper (Table 3). At the beginning of the audit period 0.8% of C&B referred patients cancelled their appointment compared to 7.0% of those referred using paper. By the end of the audit period the cancellation rates were 1.4% and 7.2% respectively.

Table 4 shows the number of "inappropriate referrals" i.e. those who were referred to a wrong clinic for some reason. At the onset of the audit period, thirteen patients out of a total of 4,385 patients referred using C&B were referred to the wrong clinic compared to only one patient out of 10,350 paper referrals. In the last quarter of the audit period 77 out of 7,263 C&B referrals were "inappropriate" compared to none out of 6,875 paper referrals.

Table 5 shows that within certain specialties such as Paediatrics there was a greater use of C&B compared to many other specialties. Even at the onset of the audit 250 (49.0%) patients were referred to the Paediatric department using C&B compared to 260 (51.0%) patients referred during the same period using paper. In the last quarter of the audit period the department of Paediatrics received 289 (68.0%) referrals through C&B while the remaining 136 (32.0%) were received through paper referrals.

19

Table 6 shows a wide variation in the number of referrals to different specialties using C&B compared to paper. While some specialties such as General Medicine registered a 100% referral using C&B, sleep studies 80.34%, Rheumatology 76.96%, and Orthopaedics 72.72% , there were other specialties where C&B was not being used at all such as Obstetrics, Trauma, Radiotherapy, Orthodontics, Care of the Elderly and Oncology services. The trend towards using C&B increased during the two year audit period.

There were differences in the referral patterns for different patient age groups and types of conditions for which the patients were referred.

Table 1; Referrals received 1st January 2008 to 31st December 2009
Appointments booked 1st January 2008 to 31st December 2009
Paper and Choose and Book split showing Total and Percentage of Referrals

		Quarter 1		Quarter 2		Quarter 3		Quarter 4		Total	
FY 2007 -2008	Choose and Book	-	- %	-	- %	-	- %	4,398	29.8%	4,398	29.8%
	Paper	-	- %	-	- %	-	- %	10,351	70.2%	10,351	70.2%
FY 2008 -2009	Choose and Book	5,149	31.5%	6,353	39.0%	6,532	40.7%	7,085	41.4%	25,119	38.2%
	Paper	11,172	68.5%	9,923	61.0%	9,505	59.3%	10,021	58.6%	40,621	61.8%
FY 2009 -2010	Choose and Book	7,561	43.4%	8,465	48.6%	7,340	51.6%	-	- %	23,366	47.6%
	Paper	9,865	56.6%	8,961	51.4%	6,875	48.4%	-	- %	25,701	52.4%

Table 2; Paper and Choose and Book split showing the percentage of DNA and Attended

		Quarter 1		Quarter 2		Quarter 3		Quarter 4		Total
		Attended	DNA	Attended	DNA	Attended	DNA	Attended	DNA	
FY 2007 -7008	Choose and Book	- %	- %	- %	- %	%	- %	95.6%	4.4%	100%
	Paper	- %	- %	- %	- %	- %	- %	94.0%	6.0%	100%
FY 2008 -2009	Choose and Book	94.6%	5.4%	94.3%	5.7%	95.0%	5.0%	93.8%	6.2%	100%
	Paper	92.7%	7.3%	92.8%	7.2%	92.2%	7.8%	91.8%	8.2%	100%
FY 2009 -2010	Choose and Book	93.1%	6.9%	92.6%	7.4%	91.8%	8.2%	- %	- %	100%
	Paper	91.9%	8.1%	90.1%	9.9%	90.4%	9.6%	- %	- %	100%

Table 3
Paper and Choose and Book split showing the percentage of Appointments with
1 or more Patient Cancellations

		Quarter 1		Quarter 2		Quarter 3		Quarter 4		Total
		Not Cancelled	Patient Cancelled	Not Cancelled	Patient Cancelled	Not Cancelled	Patient Cancelled	Not Cancelled	Patient Cancelled	
FY 2007 - 2008	Choose and Book	- %	- %	- %	- %	- %	- %	99.2%	0.8%	100%
	Paper	- %	- %	- %	- %	- %	- %	93.0%	7.0%	100%
FY 2008 - 2009	Choose and Book	98.9%	1.1%	99.0%	1.0%	99.0%	1.0%	98.7%	1.3%	100%
	Paper	91.4%	8.6%	91.1%	8.9%	92.3%	7.7%	91.4%	8.6%	100%
FY 2009 - 2010	Choose and Book	98.1%	1.9%	98.2%	1.8%	98.6%	1.4%	- %	- %	100%
	Paper	91.2%	8.8%	91.1%	8.9%	92.8%	7.2%	- %	- %	100%

Table 4: Paper and Choose and Book split showing the number of Appointments where the referred consultant was the same as the consultant at appointment

		Quarter 1		Quarter 2		Quarter 3		Quarter 4		Total
		Different	Same	Different	Same	Different	Same	Different	Same	
FY 2007 -2008	Choose and Book	-	-	-	-	-	-	13	4,385	4,398
	Paper	-	-	-	-	-	-	1	10,350	10,351
FY 2008 -2009	Choose and Book	20	5,129	44	6,309	38	6,494	47	7,038	25,119
	Paper	-	11,172	-	9,923	-	9,505	1	10,020	40,621
FY 2009 -2010	Choose and Book	40	7,521	56	8,409	77	7,263	-	-	23,366
	Paper	-	9,865	-	8,961	-	6,875	-	-	25,701

Table 5; Paper and Choose and Book split showing Total and Percentage of Referrals
Paediatrics only

		Paediatrics										Total	
		Quarter 1		Quarter 2		Quarter 3		Quarter 4					
FY 2007 – 2008	Choose and Book	-	- %	-	- %	-	- %	250	49.0%			250	49.0%
	Paper	-	- %	-	- %	-	- %	260	51.0%			260	51.0%
FY 2008 – 2009	Choose and Book	246	47.0%	260	58.7%	325	64.6%	348	65.5%			1,179	59.0%
	Paper	277	53.0%	183	41.3%	178	35.4%	183	34.5%			821	41.1%
FY 2009 – 2010	Choose and Book	343	67.4%	324	69.2%	289	68.0%	-	- %			956	68.2%
	Paper	166	32.6%	144	30.8%	136	32.0%	-	- %			446	31.8%

Table 6; Referrals received 1st January 2008 to 31st December 2009
Appointments booked 1st January 2008 to 31st December 2009
Specialty split showing Total and Percentage of Referrals

	FY 2007 - 2008				FY 2008 - 2009				FY 2009 - 2010				All Data			
	Choose and Book		Paper		Choose and Book		Paper		Choose and Book		Paper		Choose and Book		Paper	
Anaesthetics	-	0.00%	709	100.00%	-	0.00%	2,990	100.00%	-	0.00%	1,267	100.00%	-	0.00%	4,966	100.00%
Cardiology	257	37.03%	437	62.97%	1,179	41.34%	1,673	58.66%	925	42.94%	1,229	57.06%	2,361	41.42%	3,339	58.58%
Care of the Elderly	-	0.00%	192	100.00%	-	0.00%	958	100.00%	-	0.00%	642	100.00%	-	0.00%	1,792	100.00%
Clinical Haematolog	-	0.00%	66	100.00%	-	0.00%	287	100.00%	74	28.14%	189	71.86%	74	12.01%	542	87.99%
Dermatology	48	4.29%	1,070	95.71%	190	3.65%	5,010	96.35%	1,646	45.49%	1,972	54.51%	1,884	18.96%	8,052	81.04%
Dietician	-	0.00%	-	0.00%	-	0.00%	2	100.00%	-	0.00%	1	100.00%	-	0.00%	3	100.00%
Ear, Nose & Throat	916	63.52%	526	36.48%	3,692	60.60%	2,400	39.40%	2,198	52.38%	1,998	47.62%	6,806	58.02%	4,924	41.98%
Endocrinology	83	39.90%	125	60.10%	420	45.55%	502	54.45%	378	52.65%	340	47.35%	881	47.67%	967	52.33%
Gastroentrology	-	0.00%	396	100.00%	68	3.92%	1,665	96.08%	842	60.19%	557	39.81%	910	25.79%	2,618	74.21%
General Medicine	-	0.00%	-	0.00%	-	0.00%	4	100.00%	5	100.00%	-	0.00%	5	55.56%	4	44.44%
General Surgery	775	43.25%	1,017	56.75%	3,925	50.72%	3,814	49.28%	2,849	47.79%	3,112	52.21%	7,549	48.73%	7,943	51.27%
Gynaecology	536	27.07%	1,444	72.93%	2,924	40.81%	4,241	59.19%	2,168	41.68%	3,034	58.32%	5,628	39.23%	8,719	60.77%
Medical Oncology	-	0.00%	-	0.00%	-	0.00%	-	0.00%	-	0.00%	2	100.00%	-	0.00%	2	100.00%
Neurology	227	59.11%	157	40.89%	1,034	60.79%	667	39.21%	795	59.51%	541	40.49%	2,056	60.10%	1,365	39.90%
Obstetrics	-	0.00%	496	100.00%	-	0.00%	2,029	100.00%	-	0.00%	1,577	100.00%	-	0.00%	4,102	100.00%
Ophthalmology	-	0.00%	1,297	100.00%	-	0.00%	7,249	100.00%	1,741	27.65%	4,555	72.35%	1,741	11.73%	13,101	88.27%
Oral & Maxillo-Facial	81	55.10%	66	44.90%	276	51.11%	264	48.89%	217	51.79%	202	48.21%	574	51.90%	532	48.10%

Professional Project 2010

	FY 2007 - 2008				FY 2008 - 2009				FY 2009 - 2010				All Data			
	Choose and Book		Paper		Choose and Book		Paper		Choose and Book		Paper		Choose and Book		Paper	
Orthodontics	-	0.00%	2	100.00%	2	16.67%	10	83.33%	-	0.00%	3	100.00%	2	11.76%	15	88.24%
Orthopaedics	540	29.24%	1,307	70.76%	6,765	68.20%	3,155	31.80%	5,674	72.72%	2,129	27.28%	12,979	66.32%	6,591	33.68%
Paediatrics	250	49.02%	260	50.98%	1,179	58.95%	821	41.05%	956	68.19%	446	31.81%	2,385	60.97%	1,527	39.03%
Pain Management	25	37.88%	41	62.12%	171	56.07%	134	43.93%	160	54.61%	133	45.39%	356	53.61%	308	46.39%
Plastic Surgery	11	33.33%	22	66.67%	101	46.12%	118	53.88%	120	61.54%	75	38.46%	232	51.90%	215	48.10%
Radiotherapy	-	0.00%	6	100.00%	-	0.00%	24	100.00%	-	0.00%	25	100.00%	-	0.00%	55	100.00%
Respiratory	69	35.38%	126	64.62%	380	43.98%	484	56.02%	298	45.29%	360	54.71%	747	43.51%	970	56.49%
Rheumatology	262	61.36%	165	38.64%	1,164	70.21%	494	29.79%	982	76.96%	294	23.04%	2,408	71.65%	953	28.35%
Sleep Studies	27	72.97%	10	27.03%	140	56.00%	110	44.00%	94	80.34%	23	19.66%	261	64.60%	143	35.40%
Trauma	-	0.00%	144	100.00%	-	0.00%	278	100.00%	-	0.00%	244	100.00%	-	0.00%	666	100.00%
Urology	291	51.87%	270	48.13%	1,509	54.93%	1,238	45.07%	1,244	62.36%	751	37.64%	3,044	57.40%	2,259	42.60%
Total	4,398	29.82%	10,351	70.18%	25,119	38.21%	40,621	61.79%	23,366	47.62%	25,701	52.38%	52,883	40.82%	76,673	59.18%

Questionnaire Results

A total number of 250 questionnaires were electronically sent on the first of July 2010, and data was collected over a six week period till 13th August 2010; 100 of which were to General Practitioners and 150 were to Hospital Consultants. From which, 99 (40%) responses were received. Of these about 30 hospital consultants were either anaesthetist or pathologists most of whom felt that their work is not influenced in any way by C&B and hence the majority of them declined to answer. Hence the true response rate was about 43% (99/230)

The following information was collected –

1. **Age and role**

   GP's -   47 (47.5%)
   Hospital Consultants -   51 (51.5%)
   Did not answer -   1 (1%)

   Figure 3

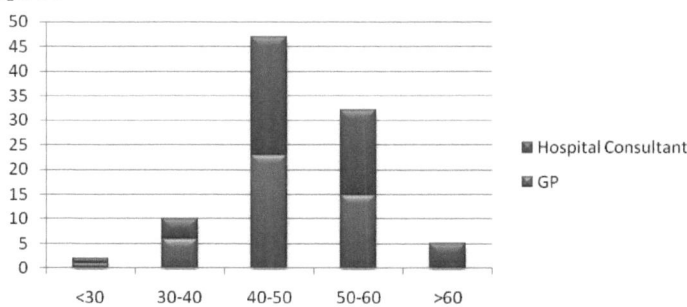

There were nearly equal numbers of GPs and hospital consultants who responded, the majority being middle aged between the ages of 40-60 years. Only five respondents were above the age of 60 and were all hospital consultants.

2. Awareness of Choose and Book

	Yes	No	Don't Know
Has it been introduced in your practice?	90.2% (83)	6.5% (6)	3.3% (3)
Do you think C&B a good idea?	38.5% (35)	49.5% (45)	2.1% (11)
Do you think C&B is delivering the Choice to patients as intended?	16.3% (15)	68.5% (63)	15.2% (14)

Figure 4:

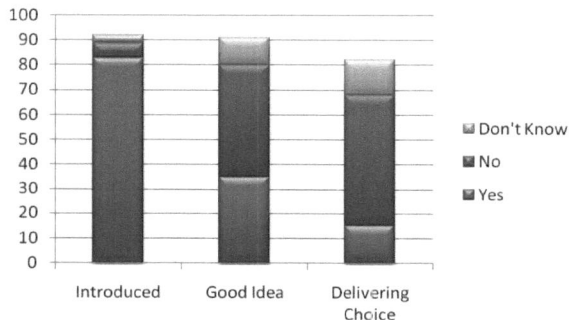

The majority of respondents did not believe C&B was delivering choice to patients. Only a 38.5% of respondents thought C&B was a good idea. It has been introduced in the majority of GP surgeries and the hospital.

3. **How familiar are you with using online services & C&B?**

	Very Familiar	Familiar	Neutral	Unfamiliar	Very Unfamiliar
How familiar are you with Using online services?	34.4% (31)	28.9% (26)	3.3% (12)	3.3% (12)	10.0% (9) 90
How familiar are you with C&B?	29.7% (27)	35.2% (32)	18.7% (17)	7.7%(7)	8.8% (8) 91

Figure 5:

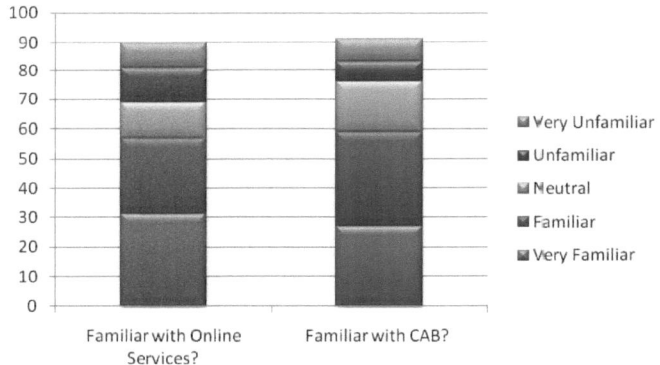

It is interesting to note that 16.5% of all respondents were either unfamiliar or very unfamiliar with C&B.

4. **How often do you think you use C&B for your patients?**

Figure 6:

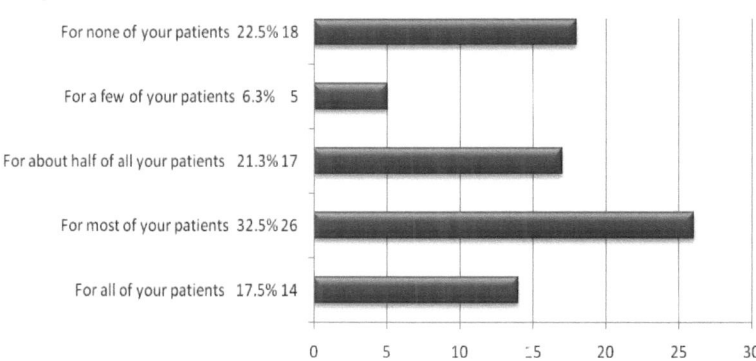

22.5% of respondents did not use C&B for any of their patients. This data was not broken down to identify who these respondents were. Some hospital specialties such as anaesthesia and pathology never get to know whether their patient has been referred to them though C&B or otherwise because they do not receive referrals directly as the patients they see have been referred via other specialties. 17.5% of respondents were using C&B for all their patients.

5. If you are a GP how many hospitals options do you offer your C&B patients?

- 1 Hospital   16.2% 6
- 2 Hospitals   **32.4% 12**
- 3 Hospitals   18.9% 7
- 4 Hospitals   **32.4% 12**

Figure 7:

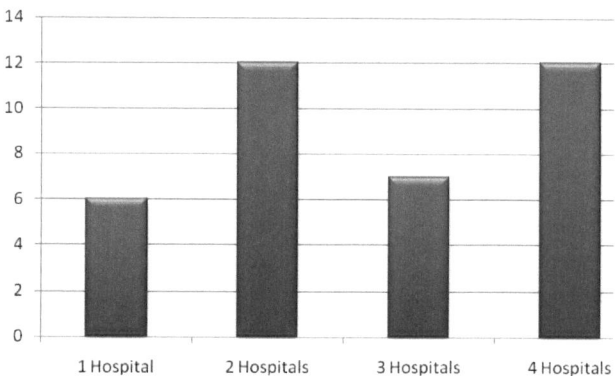

Patients should be offered at least four hospital options to choose from when using C&B but only a third of GPs offered more than three hospital options. This could be as a result of the rural setting of the local borough with only one hospital being considered by many patients and GPs as the most realist option.

6. If you are a GP based on your experience of C&B. Please answer the following:

	Excellent	Very Good	Average	Poor	Very Poor
Ease of use	5.4% (2)	21.6% (8)	**40.5% (15)**	24.3% (9)	8.1% (3)
Clinical importance of C&B	5.4% (2)	10.8% (4)	27.0% (10)	**35.1% (13)**	21.6% (8)
Convenience of use	2.7% (1)	18.9% (7)	18.9% (7)	**40.5% (15)**	18.9% (7)
Time saved	0.0% (0)	8.1% (3)	10.8% (4)	24.3% (9)	**56.8% (21)**
Training received to use	0.0% (0)	16.2% (6)	**51.4% (19)**	21.6% (8)	10.8% (4)
Functioning of Equipment	0.0% (0)	13.5% (5)	**48.6% (18)**	32.4% (12)	5.4% (2)
Reliability of equipment	0.0% (0)	10.8% (4)	**48.6% (18)**	32.4% (12)	8.1% (3)
Technical Support	5.7% (2)	11.4% (4)	**51.4% (18)**	25.7% (9)	5.7% (2)
Line Manager support	5.9% (2)	20.6% (7)	**50.0% (17)**	20.6% (7)	2.9% (1)
Team support	3.0% (1)	18.2% (6)	**57.6% (19)**	15.2% (5)	6.1% (2)
Overall experience	2.7% (1)	13.5% (5)	**37.8% (14)**	27.0% (10)	18.9% (7)

Figure 8:

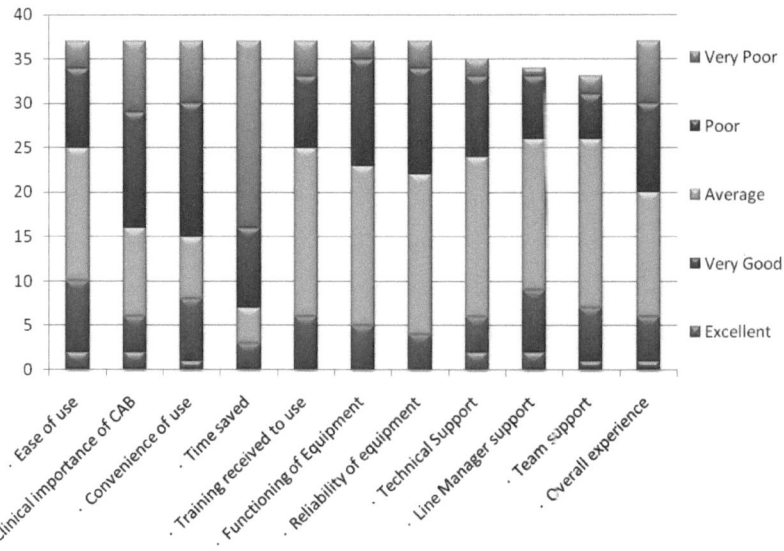

Most GPs believe that C&B takes a lot of time to use. There were no perceived benefits by the majority of GPs and consultants who rated this system as being average It was perceived by the majority to have many associated technical problems and not user friendly. More than 80% of respondents received average, poor or very poor training when it was introduced in their practices. Only 25% felt that they received very good or excellent support from their line managers.

7. If you are a hospital consultant please answer the following:

	Excellent	Very Good	Average	Poor	Very Poor
Clinical importance	0.0% (0)	6.5% (3)	45.7% (21)	32.6% (15)	**15.2% (7) 46**
Cases referred	0.0% (0)	11.1% (5)	55.6% (25)	22.2% (10)	**11.1% (5) 45**
Convenience of use	0.0% (0)	11.6% (5)	46.5% (20)	30.2% (13)	**11.6% (5) 43**
Line Manager support	0.0% (0)	14.3% (6)	59.5% (25)	14.3% (6)	**11.9% (5) 42**
Team support	0.0% (0)	19.0% (8)	52.4% (22)	16.7% (7)	**11.9% (5) 42**
Overall experience	0.0% (0)	4.4% (2)	44.4% (20)	31.1% (14)	**20.0% (9) 45**

Figure 9:

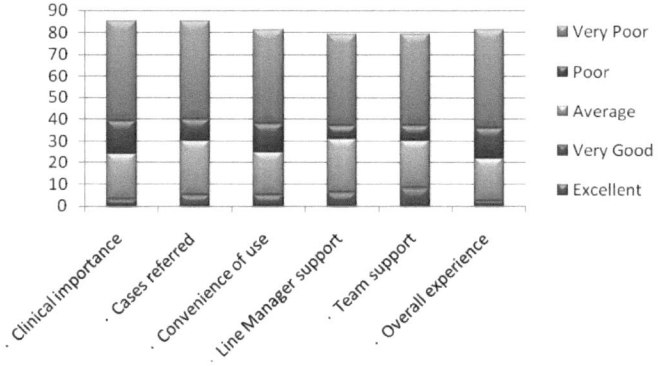

Hospital consultants did not believe C&B offered patients any special benefits. The majority thought that line manager support and team support were average. Their rating of their overall experience with the system is at best average, with 51% reporting that their experience with it is poor or very poor.

8. Regarding C&B and its benefits to your patients please answer the following:

	Strongly Agree	Agree	Neutral	Disagree	Strongly Disagree
It improves patient care	1.1% (1)	6.7% (6)	**37.8% (34)**	35.6%(32)	18.9% (17)
It improves patient attendances to appointments	1.1% (1)	29.2% (26)	**36.0% (32)**	25.8%(23)	7.9% (7)
It allows patients to have more choice in their treatment decisions	1.1% (1)	22.2% (20)	30.0% (27)	**37.8%(34)**	8.9% (8)
It improves the ability to track patient referrals	5.6% (5)	27.0% (24)	**43.8% (39)**	20.2%(18)	3.4% (3)
It reduces paperwork	2.2% (2)	13.5% (12)	15.7% (14)	**49.4%(44)**	19.1% (17)
Referrals are simpler	2.2% (2)	4.5% (4)	18.0% (16)	**51.7%(46)**	23.6% (21)
It improves the patient's experience of the healthcare system	4.5% (4)	18.2% (16)	26.1% (23)	**33.0%(29)**	18.2% (16)
It distributes appointments evenly between hospitals	0.0% (0)	8.0% (7)	32.2% (28)	**46.0%(40)**	13.8% (12)
It decreases the number of unnecessary referrals made	0.0% (0)	2.2% (2)	16.7% (15)	**51.1%(46)**	30.0% (27)
It decreases the amount of work	0.0% (0)	2.2% (2)	18.9% (17)	42.2% (38)	36.7% (33)

Figure 10:

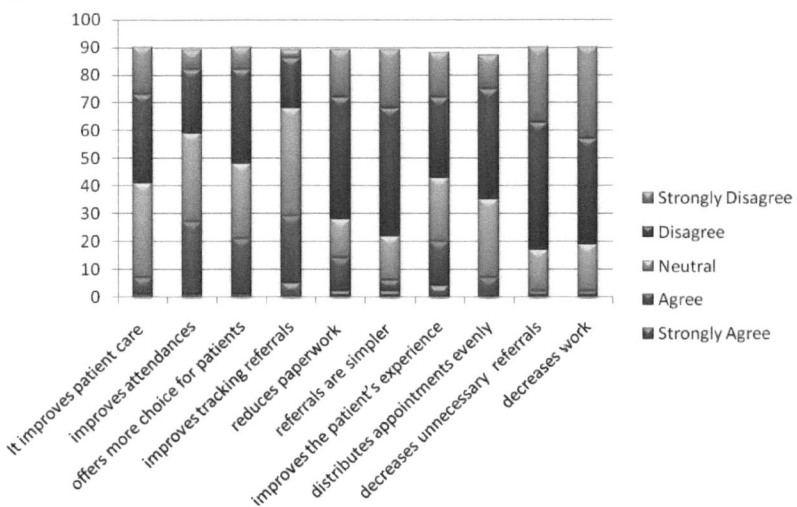

Only 7% of respondents thought that C&B improved patient care, with the majority being neutral, disagreed or strongly disagreed with this assertion. One third believed that it improved patient attendances at outpatient clinics. Only 7% believed that C&B simplified the referral process while the overwhelming majority thought that it made referral process more complicated. The majority of respondents thought C&B had no effect on providing equity of referrals to various hospitals and did not result in a decrease in unnecessary referrals. Only 2% of respondents thought it reduced workload while the overwhelming majority disagreed or strongly disagreed.

9. In your experience what do you think may be the disadvantages of C&B?

	Strongly Agree	Agree	Neutral	Disagree	Strongly Disagree
There is increased potential for confidentiality breach of patient data	5.7% (5)	17.0% (15)	**54.5% (48)**	18.2%(16)	4.5% (4)
Learning new technology is too difficult	0.0% (0)	6.7% (6)	32.6% (29)	**49.4% (44)**	11.2% (10)
There are no clearly Perceived benefits	26.7% (24)	**32.2% (29)**	17.8% (16)	20.0% (18)	3.3% (3)
There is lack of technical support when there are technical problems	3.4% (3)	27.0% (24)	**56.2% (50)**	11.2% (10)	2.2% (2)
Monetary costs associated with computerisation Including planning, purchasing training and maintenance are too high	15.9% (14)	27.3% (24)	**42.0% (37)**	12.5% (11)	2.3% (2)
Local trust doesn't have Capacity to implement & deliver C&B	3.4% (3)	12.5% (11)	**43.2% (38)**	36.4% (32)	4.5% (4)
Implementation requires you to undergo too great a change	1.1% (1)	5.7% (5)	35.2% (31)	**45.5% (40)**	12.5% (11)

Figure 11:

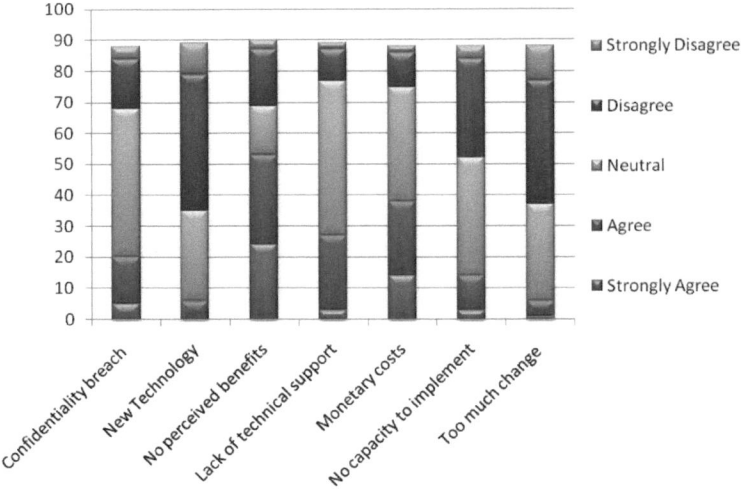

Numerous problems associated with the use of C&B have been identified, including technical issues, potential for confidentiality breaches, the fact that there appear to be no perceived benefits, the high costs involved and that this was too great a change which was implemented too quickly before all relevant clinicians were ready for it.

10. How satisfied are you with C&B & how likely are you to continue using it?

	Extremely Satisfied	Fairly Satisfied	Neutral	Fairly unsatisfied	Extremely unsatisfied
How satisfied are you with C&B?	3.3% (3)	20.0% (18)	**26.7% (24)**	23.3% (21)	**26.7% (24)**
How likely are you to continue using it?	8.4% (7)	27.7% (23)	**42.2% (35)**	10.8% (9)	10.8% (9)

Figure 12:

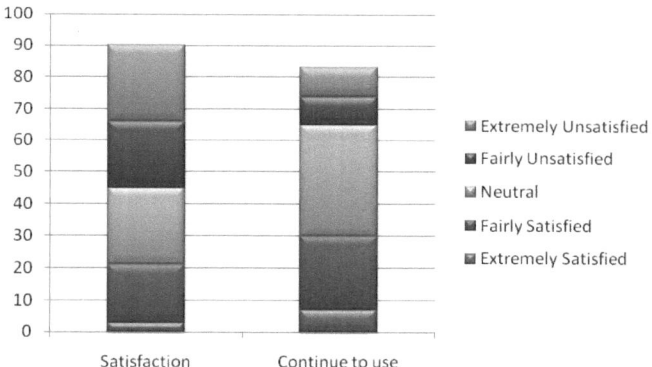

Only a quarter of respondents were satisfied with the use of C&B, with at least 50% expressing either dissatisfaction or extreme dissatisfaction. Only one third of respondents expressed a willingness to continue using it.

Table 7: Shows Emerging Themes from free text comments from GPs and Consultants:

Theme	No. Comments	As % of Total
Technical Problems	30	14.2%
Insufficient Training/Time/Information	19	9%
Increased Workload	12	5.7%
Unsuitable/Lack of belief	45	21.3%
Complex/Costly	14	6.6%
Limited Choices	62	29.4%
Hospital Issues/Cancellations/Rebooks	22	10.4%
Inappropriate Referrals	7	3.3%

Figure 13: Pie chart showing various themes

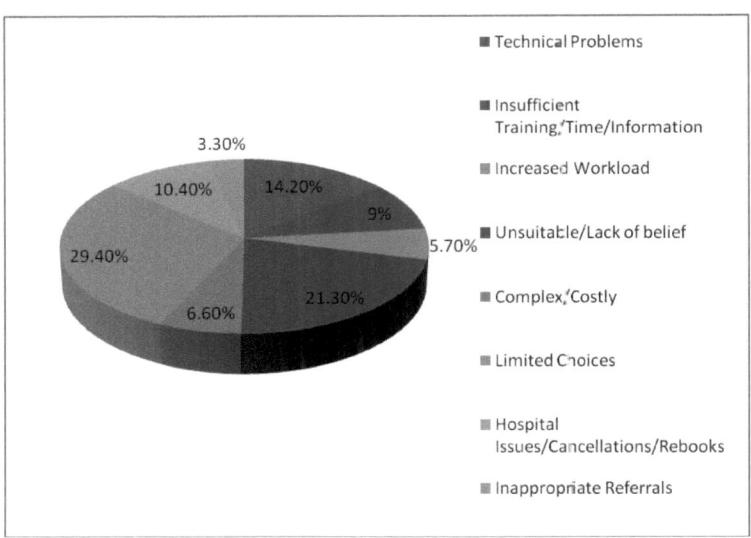

The single most frequently highlighted problem was that choice was limited in terms of the hospital itself being in a rural setting and the nearest hospital being at least 30 miles away for most patients. Hence the overwhelming number of patients preferred the local hospital. The choice of a named specialist/consultant was also often not available. Some GPs and consultants lacked belief in the system of C&B and advocated for its use to be terminated.

Technical problems such as inability to make an on line booking, patients having to wait for the hospital to call back with a specific time, and other technical issues were the third most common theme. C&B was also viewed as complicated and costly especially by the GPs. Elderly patients and ethnic minorities with a language barrier found it very difficult to use the system.

Key Findings:

- C&B is widely used within the borough at an increasing rate.

- At the end of study period 51% of all referral were through C&B. This was within the national average at the time.

- GPs vary considerably in the extent to which they actively support patient choice.

- Most patients are referred to a specialty not a named consultant

- Some local GP practices were not using C&B at all

- DNA rates were marginally better with C&B

- Patients referred using C&B showed lower cancellation rates for their appointments compared to patients referred using paper

- 'Inappropriate' referrals were higher with C&B and were re-routed internally within the trust.
  77 out of 7,263 (1.06%) C&B referrals were 'inappropriate' compared to none out of 6,875 paper referrals in the last quarter of the study period

- Some hospital specialties received higher numbers of referrals through C&B compared to others. Sleep studies (80%), Rheumatology (76.9%), Orthopaedics (72.7%), General Medicine (100%) & Paediatrics (72%) record high rates of use of C&B. Some specialties including Obstetrics, Trauma, Orthodontics, Care of the elderly and Oncology services use a different system of referral with no patients using C&B.

Questionnaire:

- 90% of respondents acknowledged that C&B had been introduced in their practices while 10%% admitted that C&B had not been introduced or the respondents did not know

- Surprisingly there was a significant number (16.5%) of GPs and Hospital consultants who are unfamiliar or very unfamiliar with the use of C&B

- Only a 38% of the respondents thought C&B was a good idea

- Only 7% of the respondents thought that C&B improved patient care.

- The majority of the respondents did not believe C&B was delivering choice to patients

- Only a third of GPs offered four or more hospital options. Two thirds of GPs reported giving patients a choice of fewer than four hospitals. 16% offered only the local hospital as an option.

- GPs were only able to select a specialty rather than a relevant named consultant

- 17.5% of respondents were using C&B for all their patients while 22.5% of respondents did not use C&B for any of their patients.
- Most GPs believe that C&B takes a lot of time to use. It was perceived by the majority of GPs to have many associated technical problems and not user friendly.
- Hospital consultants did not believe C&B offered patients any special benefits. Their rating of their overall experience with the system is at best average, with 51% reporting that their experience with it is poor or very poor.
- Only a quarter of the respondents were satisfied with the use of C&B, with at least 50% expressing either dissatisfaction or extreme dissatisfaction.
- Given a choice only one third of the respondents expressed a willingness to continue using it.
- The emerging themes from free text comments suggested that there was a lack of sufficient choice, either in the hospitals or specialists or offer in the rural setting.
- Many of the respondents reported that C&B was either unsuitable or they did not believe in it. Many of the respondents felt C&B had been imposed without their consent.
- Technical problems were impacting negatively on the successful implementation of this system.
- Short waiting times and easy access to services were considered by the GPs to be most important factors for patients.
- Certain groups of patients such as the elderly, the economically disadvantaged and ethnic minorities with a language barriers found the process very complicated and choose not to exercise choice in the majority of cases.

Chapter 5

Discussion:

At its inception, the National Health Service (NHS) was originally designed to give priority to collective needs rather than individual wants. Patient choice was not on the policy agenda within the NHS until the market oriented reforms in the 1990s (Klein, 1995). Even then it was not vigorously pursued and was mostly concerned with decisions made by general practitioner (GP) func holders contracting services from hospitals on behalf of patients (Le Grand et al, 1998).

New Labour introduced the concept of the citizen as consumer occupying a central position in its approach to modernising the public sector (Blair, 2003). By allowing patents to choose, hospitals would compete openly triggering improvements in efficiency, quality, equity and responsiveness in the NHS (DH, 2003).

However the concept of choice for the patient was largely left in the hands of GPs to implement at the point of patient consultation (DH, 2006). Some have argued that GPs are the ones who actually act as 'agents' for patients making choices on behalf of patients rather than patients making choices themselves (Le Grand et al, 1998; Williams & Rossiter, 2004). In addition patients appear to value the availability of a good GP over the opportunity to choose providers (Which, 2005). In the London Patient Choice Project, patients expressed great interest in choosing their local hospital if it meant substantial reduction in the waiting times. Where support for making choices was provided in the form of trained advisors and subsidised transport (Burge et al, 2005, Coulter et al, 2005), patients wanted to know what the comparable waiting times with other local hospitals. Reputation of the hospital was also thought to be an important factor in patient's choice. This is mirrored by the results from this evaluation where most GPs reported that patients did not wish to travel over long distances for their treatment.

Patients' ability to exercise choice was influenced by their age, gender, family obligations, socioeconomic status as shown in a study that examined patients' hypothetical preferences (Burge et al, 2005). The study found that older patients, over 60, with a low income of £10 000 and family obligations were less willing to travel. This is similar to findings in our evaluation which indicates that elderly patients and those with language barriers found it more difficult to exercise choice. Anell et al (1997) in a Swedish study, with similarities with the UK population found that younger patients in the middle class were more likely to exercise choice. Unfortunately there is evidence to suggest that patients are not sufficiently informed to make meaningful choices (Enwistle et al, 1998).

There is however, substantial evidence to suggest that patients want to exercise choice with regards to the treatment that they receive (Ford et al, 2003). Patients in England are less likely to receive the treatment choices that they require than in other countries (Shoen et al, 2004).

The results of this evaluation highlight the slow progress of implementation of the process. There are however positive signs that the process is advancing steadily towards full implementation albeit at a slow pace. This service evaluation has highlighted that the process is significantly behind schedule in terms of its implementation. The local NHS trust at the end of the audit period was receiving 51% of all its referrals through C&B. The DH schedule had anticipated that 100% of all patients would be using C&B at this stage (by the end of 2008).

Patient choice has been heralded as the driver for transforming the NHS and a means of "meeting patient expectations" (Labour Party manifesto, 2005, p. 56). However, 'Choice overload' may lead to bewilderment and anxiety, particularly for patients without access to, or the skill to understand, information to make decisions about choices on offer (Bates & Robert, 2005, 2006).

Before we can fully understand the reasons for the slow pace of implementation of C&B, we must start by analysing the key drivers of this process. What are the factors that favour rapid implementation of C&B? Patient choice is sacrosanct. In theory, most people would like to choose their GP, hospital specialist and the service they use (provider), and that this preference is increased if the patient faces a long waiting time to their local NHS provider or when the local services are poor (Enwistle et al, 1998).

What are the factors that hinder implementation of C&B? Among these factors is the lack of sufficient information given to patients at the point of delivery of the consultation. The GPs generally have insufficient time to give in detail the information required for informed choice to take place. Some GP practices have delegated the task of providing information to their secretaries and ancillary workers within the surgery. Prevailing attitudes of the medical profession and the culture within the NHS is a major contributing factor towards the slow progress to full implementation of C&B. Many patients are likely to leave the decision to the doctor who knows best. Patients believe the relationship with their consultant is important and that the

42

consultant cares for them and hence able to decide what is best for their patients (Henman et al, 2002). Many patients leave the decision to their GP with the attitude that "the doctor knows best" and wishing to avoid taking any responsibility for failure of any chosen treatment (Entwistle et al, 1998). A study by Degner & Sloan (1992) showed that six out ten patients compared to one in three members of the general public would prefer to leave treatment decisions to doctors. Patients appear to be less likely to want to exercise choice when they are in a state of uncertainty, vulnerability or distress preferring to delegate choices to a trusted medical advisor (Fortaki et al, 2006)

Providing choice for patients is likely to cost more for the NHS and any attempt at controlling such costs is liable to restrict choice as shown in the example of residential care in the UK and elsewhere (Fortaki & Boyd, 2005). Current incentives for C&B are thought to be meagre and not able to compensate for the additional time and effort required to fully implement it (Lewis, 2006).

The prevailing culture within the health sector appears to act as a hindrance to the implementation of patient choice. The London Patient Choice Project, which provided incentives for hospitals to treat more patients showed that the uptake of incentives to provide patients with choice depended on the providers' culture and capacity to implement them (Ferlie et al, 2006).

There are many factors which influence hospital performance such as competition, pricing of services, payment methods to providers, internal organisation and pre-existing culture. Furthermore, there is lack of evidence that patient choice leads to any improvement in quality of care (Fortaki et al, 2006).

Different patient groups including the elderly, female, or those with a lower education and low income, guardians of minors and family carers are less likely to select an alternative hospital to their local one for their treatment (Coulter et al, 2005).

GPs, as the primary care physicians will continue to take an active role in terms of implementing patient choice. Current Choose and Book policy assumes that GPs and the DH (via the National Institute for Health and Clinical Excellence [NICE]), will play a role in framing the choices which patients are offered. Patient choice hence is limited to the options left after the framing process (DH, Choose & Book, 2004).

Choice for patients will invariably create a need for additional resources for providers to enable them to offer all the relevant treatment options which are potentially available. The cost of these additional resources is uncertain. In the end providers may then end up choosing the patients that they can treat if they cannot provide the whole range of treatment options. There is a risk that patients may come into conflict with NICE by choosing options which are not considered cost effective or of proven efficacy. There have been already examples of this in the media with patients suing trusts for not providing certain treatments which patients wanted offered.

Fotaki et al (2008) make the assertion that, although patients may themselves make limited use of choices, the existence of choice may, in theory, stimulate providers to improve quality of care. Patients, however, want to be more involved in individual decisions about their own treatment, and generally participate much less in these decisions than they would wish. Patients consider access to a good local hospital to be more appropriate than having more hospitals from which to choose (Which, 2005).

C&B has met with significant scepticism from clinicians. It has provided a formidable challenge to both primary and secondary care. Some GPs feel that choice for patients is being used to influence quality and equity issues rather between hospitals rather than to benefit the patient themselves. Enthusiasts argue that patient choice forces hospitals and trusts to be more responsive to patients needs. Many clinicians have found the ethical, clinical and technological elements which influence their attitude, linking these frustrations with their general sense of a loss of professional status and power (Walford 2006). As demonstrated in this review many practitioners find C&B to be time consuming and it increases their workload. GPs have expressed concerns about confidentiality breaches using C&B (BBC News, 2006).

Patient choice requires accurate data to be available. Dr Foster has demonstrated that outcome data can be presented in a way patients can understand, although this has sometimes caused much irritation to clinicians and trusts alike. The Care Quality Commission is taking a key role to publish validated comparative data about various hospitals and clinical services.

Patients generally want to be seen as quickly as possible. Patients may leave the GP surgery with a triple uncertainty. Firstly the fact that they need to see a specialist indicates that there could be a serious underlying illness. Secondly the fact that they need to visit a hospital but do not know which one and when. Thirdly that they know little or nothing about the specialist they will see. C&B helps alleviate some of these concerns. Using the C&B IT application the GP can automatically construct a letter containing the key details and the reason for the referral. The patient also has the extra option of making the booking by telephone or through the internet. C&B provides direct booking, communication systems which are secure, clear, flexible reassuring the patient at the same time. These appointments can also be tracked down quickly on line by the GP and patient.

Despite the theoretical advantages of C&B, there is a 'culture' that exists within the NHS that doctors generally know what is good for the patients and that they are the best guardians of how the system should be managed for the good of the patients. This in part could be the reason of the slow implementation of C&B where the patient decides how and where they may be treated. There is a culture of resistance from the medical profession to the increasing marketisation of the NHS health care. There is a need for change to occur for full implementation of C&B to take effect. Change can be defined as a planned or unplanned response of an organization to pressure (Dalziel & Schoonover, 1988). Change may result from the outside environment in the form of new competition, new social values, or new business practices. In all its forms, change creates opportunities and vulnerabilities.

The original meaning of 'culture' is something that is cultivated such as crops. Williams (1983) uses it in social phenomena to signify processes of human socialisation through institutions such as family, community, religion and education. It was not until 1979 that the phrase 'organisational culture' was coined (Pettigrew, 1979), and until the 1980s that the topic emerged as a distinct entity in mainstream management thought. It was then thought that organisational culture played an important role in influencing employee motivation and organisational performance. Smircich (1983) defines culture as the beliefs and/ or values that organisation members have in common. It is seen as "the way things get done here" or patterns of shared assumptions that have been reinforced by their apparent success in solving organisational problems (Schein 1995). This approach treats culture as a variable or attribute, alongside others such as the organisation's technology, business strategy and other important relevant factors. The implication of this approach is that culture can be viewed as an attribute that can be taught and subject to manipulation or that it can be 're-engineered' for management purposes to 'fit' the organisation's external environment. This concept contrasts the alternative view as something that the organisation 'is' (Morgan, 2006). This latter approach implies the existence of fewer levers by which management might secure change, since the entire organisation is seen as a cultural system in itself.

Some elements within culture are more deeply embedded in organisations and therefore more difficult to change. Schein (1985) distinguishes between artefacts, values and basic assumptions. Artefacts form the most visible 'surface' level of an organisation's culture, including the physical environment, products, technology, overt behaviour and the use language and other symbolic forms. Values underlie and influence behaviour 'what ought to be done' rather than 'what is', and therefore include ethical and ideological positions. Finally, basic assumptions are the deepest level of an organisation's culture, including causal and normative beliefs that have become internalised by members that it is now a subconscious part of their activities.

Table 8: Showing Five Models of Organisational Culture Change (Scott et al, 2003)

Models:

- Lundberg's model, based on earlier learning cycle models of organisational change; emphasises external environmental factors as well as internal characteristics of organisations
- Dyer's model, posits that the perception of crisis in conjunction with a leadership change are required for culture change to occur
- Schein's model, based on a simple life-cycle framework; posits that different culture change mechanisms are associated with different stages in an organisation's development
- Gagliardi's model, suggests that only incremental culture change can properly be described as a form of organisational change
- A composite model based on the ideas of Lewin, Beyer and Trice, and Isabella; provides some insights into the microprocesses of culture.

It is beyond the scope of this project to review all these models but I will focus primarily on Lungberg's model which is based on the assumption that for culture change to occur several internal and external conditions must be in place. Internal permitting conditions that facilitate change are; a) sufficient change resources (e.g. finance, managerial time, and commitment), b) system readiness (a shared assumption that organisation members support change), c) coordinative and integrative mechanisms that allow communication and control and d) a stable leadership group with awareness, vision, power and communication skills to lead the desired culture change. There are four types of precipitating pressures that influence the likeliness of change which have been identified. The first is a typical performance related demand (e.g. incentives to improve performance). The second type are stakeholder pressures (including the public, pressure groups and external regulators, etc). The third type are pressures arising from rapid organisational growth or contraction. The forth type of pressure is a perception of crisis (e.g. financial losses or large debts). Lungberg's model proposes one further condition which is needed before cultural change can take place, namely a triggering event. This event could take the form of an environmental disaster or opportunity, internal revolutions or management crisis.

For any cultural change to be successful there needs to be a strategy which should be implemented through action plans. Such a change should contain three important factors; the pace of change (quick or slow paced), the scope of change (how radical?), and the time span (over how long should the change be managed?)

In the context of C&B findings from this evaluation it is clear that employing Lungberg's proposed action planning would resolve some of the problems the system is facing. Three particular forms of action planning are needed; a) inducement action plans that strengthen organisational preparedness for change, b)management action plans that enable members to re-imagine the existing culture in line with the culture change strategy and c)stabilising action plans reinforcing the changes and ensure their longevity.

Unfortunately Lungberg's model fails to address the political forces (doctor- managerial tensions) within organisations, or recognise the influence of key individuals and groups in facilitating or resisting culture change (Scott et al 2003).

Dyer's model offers a different perspective to cultural change. In this model a crisis triggers a need for change. This is usually initiated by an adverse event, which creates a perception of crisis that organisational members believe cannot be resolved thorough the use of existing strategies and practices. In healthcare organisations, examples of such crises could arise from a loss of public confidence caused by a high profile failure in professional or clinical practice. This breakdown is necessary to make way for a new culture. Crisis affecting the old leadership creates way for new leadership with unique opportunities to change the existing culture within the organisation. By bringing and embedding new artefacts, perspectives, values, and assumptions into the organisation. (Dyer, 1985)

Schein (2005) defines organisational culture by three levels; artefacts, values, and assumptions. Artefacts are things that we can see, hear and sense when we enter an organisation. Values are how the organisation does what it does. Assumptions are values that have become embedded in the culture are taken for granted. Cultural change can be brought about by looking at discrepancies between artefacts and espoused values. We should try to uncover those assumptions that explain these discrepancies. Planned change and organisational development involves facilitating culture change by analysing and bringing to the surface the values and assumptions of the dominant culture and subcultures.

Garliardi's concept of cultural change advocated that the change should occur incrementally, not radically (Garliardi 1986). Garliardi argues that the need for large scale change is rarely perceived by those deeply involved in its culture and more likely to be seen by members of counter-cultures or outsiders. Culture change hence requires a change in leadership, from outside the dominant culture.

Patient choice is here to stay and the NHS should freely embrace it. The recently published white paper, 'Equity and Excellence', by the DH, (2010) aims to further strengthen the principle that patient empowerment, facilitated by information and choice of health provider is paramount. It seeks to 'free the provider market and promote greater choice'. It proposes the introduction of increasingly robust regulations directed towards internationally comparable quality outcomes and the effective use of resources. A subsequent document 'Transparency in Outcomes –A Framework for the NHS', states that nationally the focus will be on outcomes rather than structure and process (DH, 2010).

Recommendations:

- In a rural setting the need to provide patients with access to other healthcare providers should be recognised and resourced.
- Maintaining a good local hospital with a good reputation and short waiting times is vitally important for the local population.
- GPs need extra resources to allow patients to make choices especially to offer patients access to other providers through providing transport for patients.
- The language used to patients must be changed. Language of decisions and consequences not just 'choices'
- Patients should be actively encouraged to 'think actively' during consultation to facilitate better decision making.
- Higher levels of intervention such as decision aids and motivational interviewing should be employed
- There needs to be a culture change within the NHS where the patient is allowed to have free choice.
- The local hospital must provide accurate data on its services and outcomes.
- Choose and Book system should include the option to refer to a named consultant.
- There is a need to develop supporting services, such as choice advisers or health advisory centres, to support patient choice.
- GPs and hospital consultants need to work more closely together and assist each other in offering patient choice.

48

- More effort needs to be put into convincing the 'sceptic' GPs and hospital consultants about the benefits of C&B for their patients.
- GPs' job plans should be cognisant of the extra time required to implement C&B.
- Local health service provision should be made more effective and efficient.

Next Step:

- GPs and consultants need to strengthen existing links and sharing of information through a combined GP-/consultant forum so that GPs are better informed about what services the local provider can offer. Barriers between GPs and Hospital consultants should be broken. There should be shared values and open communication between the two groups.
- Strong leadership is required within the local medical fraternity to guide members through culture change which allows patient choice to take effect within the local NHS. This role could be taken by the more influential members of the GP and consultant communities to champion a culture change to put patients at the heart of everything. These leaders should be chosen by the local medical professionals, not a top to bottom implementation.
- The local trust must provide GPs with accurate data on specialists/consultants available and what service they provide
- Patient choice advisory service needs to be established in the form of choice information centres for patients.

Conclusion:

Medical professionals as frontline providers of services in the NHS need to embrace the principle of "patient choice" as paramount. There is a need for a change in culture with n the NHS for C&B to be implemented at a more rapid pace. Although C&B was "imposed" by the DH, local health professionals must begin to regard C&B as their own and set their own agenda of implementing it fully It is important that GPs encourage their patients to make reasoned healthcare decisions that are informed by an evaluation of the options rather than by a simple preference for choice. Patient training centres need to be established to inform patients about their choices and greater resources put in place to allow patients to take up various options.

References:

Anell A, Rose´n P, Hjortsberg C, (1997). Choice and participation in the health services: a survey of preferences among Swedish residents. *Health Pol;40:157–68*

Appleby J, Alvarez A. (2005) Public Responses to NHS Reform. *In British Social Attitudes Survey 22nd Report, 'Two terms of Labour: the public's reaction' Volume chapter 5. Edited by: Park et al. London, Sage*

Bate P, Robert G, (2005). Choice. *BMJ 331:1488-9.*

Bate P, Robert G, (2006). 'Build it and they will come' – or will they? Choice, policy paradoxes and the case of the NHS treatment centres. *Policy & Politics 34:651-672.*

BBC News, (2006). *GPs dissatisfied with IT system. London.* [http://news.bbc.co.uk/go/pr/fr/-/1/hi/health/5028762.stm] (Accessed 25th August 2010)

Bentley, J and Fletcher D (2007) Choosing and using: patient choice in 'Choose and Book'. *British Journal of Community Nursing, vol./is. 12/12 (558-562)*

Blair A, (2003). We must not waste this precious period of power. *Speech given at South Camden Community College, 23 January 2003.* See www.labour.org.uk/tbsocialjustice

Brennan S (2005). NHS IT project: the biggest computer programme in the world . .ever! *Oxford: Radcliffe Medical Press.*

Bryant, L (2007). The lure of 'patient choice'. *British Journal of General Practice 57: 822-826*

Burge P, Devlin N, Appleby J, Rohr C, Grant J, (2005). London Patient Choice Project evaluation. A model of patients' choices of hospital from stated and revealed preference choice data. *Cambridge: RAND Europe.*

Coiera EW, (2007). Lessons from the NHS National Programme for IT. *MJA 186:3-4*

Coombes R, (2006). Patients get four choices for NHS treatments. *BMJ ;332: 8*

Coulter A (2003). Engaging patients and citizens. In: Leatherman S, Sutherland K (eds), The quest for quality in the NHS. *London: The Nuffield Trust,*

Coulter A, Le Maistre N, Henderson L, (2005). Patients' experience of choosing where to undergo surgical treatment. Evaluation of the London Patient Choice scheme. *Oxford: Picker Institute.*

Coulter A, Magee H (2003). The European Patient of the Future Maidenhead. *Open University Press*

Dalziel MM, Schoonover SC, (1988). Changing Ways - A Practical Tool For Implementing Change Within Organizations. AMACON a division American Management Association, 135 W. 50th Street, *New York, New York.*

Degner LF, Sloan JA, (1992). Decision making during serious illness: What role do patients really want to play? *J Clin Epidemiol;45:941–50*

Department of Health *(2003).* Building on the Best: *Choice, Responsiveness and Equity in the NHS. London.*

Department of Health (2003). Developing choice, responsiveness and equity in health and social care "Fair for all and personal to you" a national consultation exercise – *letter. London*

Department of Health (2004). The NHS improvement plan: putting people at the heart of public services. *London: DH. Cm 6268.*

Department of Health (2006). *Choice at Referral: Guidance Framework for 2006/2007. London.*

Department of Health (2006). Patient Choice. *London.*

Department of Health (DH), (2003). Building on the best: cho ce, responsiveness and equity in the NHS. *London: Department of Health.*

Department of Health, (2004). Choose and Book. London: Department of Health. See http://www. chooseandbook.nhs.uk/

Department of Health, (2008). Introduction of Free Choice policy. http://www.dh.gov.uk/en/Publicationsandstatistics/Lettersandcirculars/Dearcolleagueletters/DH_083697 (Accessed 9th August 2010)

Department of Health, (2010). Equity and excellence: Liberating the NHS. *White Paper.*

Department of Health, (2010). *Transparency in Outcomes —A Framework for the NHS.* http://www.dh.gov.uk/en/Consultations/Liveconsultations/DH_117583 (Accessed 27th August 2010)

Dyer WG, (1985). The cycle of cultural evolution in organizaticns. Control of the Corporate Culture. *San Francisco: Josey-Bass*

Entwistle VA, Sheldon TA, Sowden A, Watt IS, (1998). Evidence-informed patient choice. *Int J Tech Assess Health Care;14:212–25*

Ferlie E, Freeman G, McDonnell J, Petsoulas C, Rundle-Smith S, (2006). Introducing choice in the public services: some supply side issues. *Publ Money Manag;26:62–72*

Ford S, Schofield T, Hope T, (2003). Are patients' decision-making preferences being met? *Health Expectations;6:72–80*

Fotaki M, Boyd A, (2005). From Plan to Market: a comparison of health and old age care policies in the UK and Sweden. *Publ Money Manag;25:237–43*

Fotaki M, Boyd A, Smith L, et al (2006). Patient choice and the organisation and delivery of health services: scoping review. A report to the NHS Service Delivery and Organisation (NCCSDO). *London: SDO.* See www.sdo.lshtm.ac.uk/files/project/80-final-report.pdf (Accessed 20th August 2010)

Glaser BG, Strauss AL (1967). The discovery of grounded theory: strategies for qualitative research. *New York: Aldine de Gruyter.*

Green J, McDowall Z, Potts WWH (2008). Does Choose and Book fail to deliver the expected choice of patients? A survey of patients' experience of outpatient appointment booking. *BMC Medical Informatics and Decision Making;8:36.*

Hendy J, Reeves BC, Fulop N, et al (2005). Challenges to irrplementing the national programme for information technology (NPfIT): a qualitative study. *BMJ; 331: 331-336.*

Henman MJ, Butow PN, Brown RF, Boyle F, Tattersall MHN, (2002). Lay constructions of decision-making in cancer. *Psycho-Oncol;11:295–306*

http://www.dh.gov.uk/en/Publicationsandstatistics/Publications/PublicationsPolicyAndGuidance/DH_117353 [Cm7881]. (Accessed 27th August 2010)

Hutt R, Rosen R, Florin D, (2006). An Anatomy of GP Referral Decisions A qualitative study of GPs' views on their role in supporting patient choice. *Kings Fund.*

Klein R (1995). The new politics of the NHS. London: Routledge

Lakhani M, Baker M (2006). Good General Practitioners will continue to be essential. *BMJ ;332:41-43*

Le Grand J, Mays N, Dixon J. Conclusions. In: Le Grand J, Mays N, Mulligan JA, eds (1998). Learning From the NHS Internal Market. A review of the evidence. *London: Kings Fund Publishing:117–34*

Lewis D M (2006). Patients get four choices for NHS treatments. Choose and book has not left the station. *BMJ ;332:180*

M Rashid, L Abeysundra, A Mohd-Isa et al (2007). Two years and £196 million later: where is choose and book? *Informatics in Primary Care 15:111–19*

Miles MB, (1979). Qualitative data as an attractive nuisance- the problem of analysis. *Adm Sci Q 24: 590-601*

Modayil P C, Hornigold R, Glore R J, Bowder D A, (2009); Patients' attendance at clinics is worse with choose and book. *BMJ;338:b396*

Morgan G, (2006). Images of Organisation. *Sage Publications Inc.*

National Health Service. *NHS in England. Choosing your hospital.* http://www.nhs.uk/England/Choice/ (Accessed 20th August 2010).

NHS Direct website. http://www.chooseandbook.nhs.uk/patents/whatiscab (Accessed 20th August 2010)

NHS Executive, (1997). R&D in Primary Care: national working group report. *Leeds*

NICE, (2002), Principles for Best Practice in Clinical Audit 2002

Oates J (2007). Doctors slam Choose and Book. Choose and Book unfit for purpose. *Weekly Computer; 27TH June 2007*

Pettigrew AM, (1979). On Studying Organisational Culture. *Administrative Science Quarterly 24:570*

Pothier DD, Awad Z, Tierney P. (2006). 'Choose and Book' in ENT: the GP perspective. *J Laryngol Otol;120:222-5.*

Rabiei R, Bath PA, Hutchinson A, Burke D. (2009). The National Programme for IT in England: clinicians' views on the impact of the Choose and Book service. *Health Informatics J;15:167-78*

Schein EM, (1985); How culture forms, develops and changes. Gaining control of the corporate culture. *San Fransisco: Jossey-Bass*

Schoen C, Osborn R, Huynh PT, et al, (2004). Primary care and health system performance: adults' experiences in five countries. *Health Aff;23:89–99*

Schwartz B, (2004). The paradox of choice: why more is less. *New York: Harper Collins.*

Scott T, Mannion R, Davies H, Marshall M, (2003). The Quantitative Measurement of Organizational Culture in Health Care: A Review of the Available Instruments. *Health Services Research 38:923-945*

Smircich L, (1983). Concept of Culture and Organisational Analysis. *Administrative Science Quarterly 28:339-358*

The Labour Party (2005). *Britain Forward Not Back: The Labour Party Manifesto 2005. London.*

Walford S, (2006). Choose and Book. *Clin Med 6:473–6*

Which?, (2005). *Choices Omnibus Survey. London.*

Which?, (2005); Which choice? Health. London: *Which?, 2005*

Williams J, Rossiter A, (2004). Choice: the evidence. The operation of choice systems in practice: national and international evidence. London: *The Social Market Foundation.*

Williams R (1983). Culture in society, 1780-1950. *Columbia University Press.*

Wood J. (2006). Patients get four choices for NHS treatments: Choose and book will hinder development of good outpatient services. *BMJ;332:180*

APPENDIX 1

Choose and Book Report 2010

Introduction

Choose and Book and Patient Choice.

The NHS Constitution, published on 21 January 2009, established a new right to choice and to information to support that choice. Choose and Book provides the perfect tool to ensure that referrers have up to date and relevant information to enable patients to access their right to choice.

From April 2008, all patients registered with an English GP were given the right to choose from any NHS funded provider following a referral to a hospital consultant. The only exceptions being cases requiring speed of access, such as suspected cancer and chest pains, in addition to maternity and mental health services.

In April 2009 that right to choice was written into the NHS Constitution. Patients have a legal right to choose where (from any NHS funded provider in England) and when (from published dates and times) they wish to be seen when referred for a first outpatient appointment in a consultant lead service.

Results from patient choice surveys show the key factors influencing patients in their choice are:

- accessibility
- cleanliness
- reputation
- waiting times
- quality of care

Choose and Book is a national electronic referral service that lists the services of all providers in England with up-to-date information about conditions treated, exceptions and waiting times to enable referrers to assist their patients in making an informed choice of place, date and time for their first outpatient appointment in a hospital or clinic. It allows patients to choose a hospital or clinic and book an appointment with a specialist. [1]

Overview

Benefits for Patients

- Patients can choose any hospital in England funded by the NHS (this includes NHS hospitals and some independent hospitals).
- Patients can also choose their preferred date and time from the available appointments offered by the hospital provider.
- Patients experience greater convenience and certainty. With Choose and Book, the choice is theirs.
- There is less chance that information will get lost in the post because more correspondence takes place through computers.
- Patients can check the status of their referral and change or cancel appoints easily over the phone or on the internet.
- Benefits to NHS Staff and Clinicians
- GPs can search for services that are available for different conditions and get information on waiting times whilst with the patient.
- Choose and Book helps improve the communication between primary and secondary care and ensures that the patient's journey through the system is transparent and effectively managed.
- Choose and Book's Advice and Guidance facility offers GPs the opportunity to discuss cases electronically with consultants in hospitals, helping to ensure that patients do actually need a referral and, if so, that they are booked into the correct clinic.
- GPs and practice staff see a reduction in the amount of time spent on the paper chase and bureaucracy associated with existing referral processes.
- Did Not Attends (DNAs) have reduced at a number of trusts, because patients have been more involved in deciding where and when they will be seen by a consultant or specialist.
- By reducing the time spent waiting to receive their first outpatient appointment, Choose and Book will help measure and manage the 18 weeks pathway for patients.

Primary care clinicians

What does Choose and Book mean for a Primary Care Clinician?

- Able to book patients into available appointment slots for services that have been locally commissioned or which are available across the NHS through Free Choice.
- Continue to use current Primary care systems - many of these systems are Choose and Book service compliant so when it is decided to make a referral, it can make a seamless transition into the Choose and Book service. The patient's name, NHS number etc are transferred through to the Choose and Book service automatically.
- If there is no practice system at all, access to the Choose and Book service can directly from a desktop computer via a web interface.
- Choose and Book provides a Directory of Services enabling to search for and review available services.
- The opportunity to view Booking guidance to help in the decision making process if required.

Advantages for Primary care clinicians

- Using the advice and guidance capability from within Choose and Book gives the opportunity for GPs to discuss cases electronically with consultants in hospitals, often helping to ensure that patients do actually need a referral and if so are booked into the correct clinic (advice and guidance facility)
- Patients whose appointments are booked electronically no longer need to make follow up visits to the practice to find out what has happened to their referral
- Possible reduction in secretarial time with less time spent chasing up appointments
- A full directory of all services available
- Immediate access to services with shortest waiting times
- Can get an appointment for patients 'on-line'

- Booking guidance is available to ensure patients are seen in the most appropriate clinics
- The ability to track referrals through the referral pathways and generate a work list to avoid lost letters.

Secondary care clinicians

How does Choose and Book help a Secondary Care Clinician?

- A Secondary care clinician (eg hospital consultant) will have greater certainty that the right patients will be booked into clinics - and that patients will attend their appointments.
- Each trust will create a directory of services showing all of the services they provide. Clinicians are able to input into that process to ensure that the directory accurately reflects your services and that pertinent information is available to all clinicians who refer to the services.
- In order to access Choose and Book your trust will need to allocate you an NHS smartcard. They will also need to make sure the necessary hardware and software is available in both the clinical and office environment.
- Finally Clinicians, will need to receive training from your trust in order to fully utilise the functionality of the application.

Advantages for Secondary care clinicians

- It reduces the number of patients who don't turn up for appointments at hospital (DNAs)
- Consultants in Secondary Care have found that using the Advice and Guidance function facilitates dialogue with GPs, helping to ensure patients are booked into the correct clinic
- Advice and Guidance may also reduce face to face outpatient appointments
- Ability to reject referrals if not appropriate for a particular clinic
- All referrals will be legible and remove the need for GPs to be contacted for clarification
- An opportunity to manage clinic workload
- Appointment reminders
- Dispense with the need for paper referrals and the risk associated with losing them - a secure and certain way of referral
- The ability to review referrals in any clinical setting and whenever the clinician has time
- Through workgroups, allow other clinicians to review referrals, eg, when on holiday.

Training Overview

With the implementation and ongoing enhancement of a system affecting all areas of the NHS, training and education are essential to support successful delivery.

The Choose and Book National Training team is responsible for a number of areas as outlined below:

- Produce the National Choose and Book Training Strategy detailing the approach to be taken by the Team for the development and delivery of Training.
- Work with the SHA Education Training and Development (ETD) colleagues to ensure the strategic direction of training reflects the requirements of the Choose and Book community.
- Undertake regular Training Needs Analysis.
- Deliver Train the Trainer courses in Primary and Secondary care to trainers and facilitators across the NHS community.
- Develop documentation to support the NHS Community
- Ensure user knowledge of functionality is maintained following a Choose and Book release.
- Maintain training tools e.g. the Demonstration Environment and Choose and Book Unplugged to ensure they reflect current functionality,
- Produce presentations and Lesson Plans to support trainers and facilitators for delivery of a consistent training message.
- Facilitate the Choose and Book Training Forum.
- Educate end-users through regular communication updates via the website or the communications tool.
- Produce reports to reflect the training undertaken from a national level.
- Evaluate each course delivered by the National Training Team and action where necessary.

Training Principles

There are a number of key principles that underpin the training provision from the Choose and Book National Training team.

- Employing various methods of instruction
- Chalk and talk
- Group discussions
- Demonstrations
- Exercises
- Learning through using.

Throughout the training courses, delegates are given ample opportunity to use the system 'hands on' to reinforce their knowledge. This allows them to experiment with the system and confirm their understanding.

Having completed a course, delegates are required to complete a written Assessment to confirm their understanding of the subject matter. [1]

Aims and Objectives

This audit is aimed to evaluate the use of the Choose and Book referral system that is used by the Hospital Consultants, and General Practitioners in the local Primary Care Service and measured against the Choose and Book Standards.

Criteria and Standards

Using the aims and standards set out by the Choose and Book service, and by obtaining views and feedback from healthcare professionals it is hoped to identify areas of poor compliance and ascertain how to improve on user and patient experience.

Sample and Methodology

A simple questionnaire was designed using an online survey software[2]. This was disseminated electronically to all local general practitioners and hospital consultants to obtain data and feedback for analysis.

Once responses were received, the data was downloaded for analysis with assistance from the Trust's Clinical Audit Department.

Results
-See tables of results and histograms

Choose and Book – *Comments from respondents*

- *When it works it works well, but often it does not work. I recently found out that up to 40% of appointments are subsequently rebooked! It also relies on the directories being correctly put on by the hospital trust.*

- *Does not offer real choice, nor does it seem easy to use. Many appts made through choose and book are altered once the consultant has read the letter.*

- *Crazy system; never relevant; often wont work>frustration and time wasting; hospital data usually inaccurate, so misleading patients=poor choice (never relevant around here; rural location - only one true provider; choice here=fiction; choice might be real in London = oversupply*

- *I have not answered the first question because it is too black and white. The principle of patients having a choice is a good one but in actual fact in my experience the vast majority of our patients merely want to go to the local hospital in a timely manner. Its function therefore does not meet a local demand. More importantly the fact the system is entirely administratively led has led to the situation locally where the consultants do not read the referral letters before the patient attends outpatients. This removes a key safety net allowed by the old system whereby consultants could altered a referral priority if the clinical situation warranted it. The system is medico-legally unsafe and not in the best interests of patients.*

- *Too restrictive - in terms of highlighting needs of individual patients to specialist clinicians (not administrators) however it does allow pt's choice and spreads the workload.*

- *I think in this area it is a huge waste of money as the majority of patients opt to go to ..... Patients appreciate being able to book an appt in the Drs consulting room, however all too often this has to be rearranged. most patients prefer to go to the local hospital, choice is not the key feature, it has helped with booking appt on line, so more convenient to patients and clearer. appt times at some specialities still take too long though.*

- *Patients almost without exception choose a local hospital. Their ultimate decision remains unchanged compared to pre C+B but we have a better idea of which community hospitals have which clinics.*

- *Doesnt always result in shorter waiting times. Not always appropriate for patients to travel.*

- *good idea but poorly executed*

- *personal and patient experience - choice is very restricted. Not enough information given to patients for informed choice. Elderly patients (i.e. most of the needy sick) find this difficult or impossible to negotiate*

- *Patients don't want choice, they want to be seen locally and quickly!*

- *Less choice as unable refer to a specific consultant. In a place like .....it is irrelevant as the next nearest |hospital is 30 miles away - very few of my patients want to travel that far*

- *gives more choice re day and time but may not be the correct specialist*

- *most patients use their local hospital regardless*

- *Services constantly changing and up to date information is not available in a single easily accessible place.*

- *Some patients lack transport resources to choose anything other than their nearest hospital.*

- *except in a town like Swindon very few people want to travel further than ...... and take up other choices*

- *It is impossible to say whether a good idea or not in one word- yes as it give patients control of when their appt will be. no as it removes ability to refer to specific consultants/ clinics*

- *to avoid wasting valuable GP time we delegate admin tasks to appropriately trained admin staff - in this case Mandy our very capable secretary. I have a smartcard to access choose'n'book, it hasn't worked for at least 2 years, I haven't missed it (and I'm PBC lead for the practice)*

- *Time consuming in consultations; cannot select consultant; 99% Swindon patients prefer to be seen in .....*

- *Most patients still prefer to travel to local hospital was it wise to introduce so time consuming a system for us gps for a tiny minority?*

- *patients want to be able to request a specific consultant*

- *Patients are often confused. They can choose time and day but not specialty interest or even a female/male consultant.*

- *Our patients mostly want the local hospital......... anyway. If they want an alternative it is often not available. If they want a consultant choice it is also not easy*

- *Prevents patients being referred to correct consultant*

- *Most patients choose not to exercise choice*

- *Most want a swift and good service from the local hospital and few want to go further afield. Many are confused by the choices and the process is disruptive to the consultation. When other hospitals are selected eg....... the patients are often then unhappy with the need to attend hospitals such as..... for investigations as this is not clear in the initial selection process*

- *As we have only one main local provider the idea of choice to 90% of patients if a falsehood;however the other 0% at least have the possibility raised*

- *There is no choice of consultant. We are not able to choose services that get near to breaching a wait list target as they are removed from the choice list intermittently.*

- *The patient is only able to choose based on time to consult. they cannot choose to specifically see a consultant, in a cons named clinic for example*

- *The choice was available before Choose and Book, the system has actually restricted choice in some ways, as well as wasting huge amounts of our time*

- *GP's don't know name of consultant when booking "Tuesday morning"*

- *98% of my patients choose the local district general hospital*

- *Mostly does, sometimes can't ref to some depts. Our patients aren't really fussed about choice, they just want to go to the local hospital*

- *It's not at all useful. Patients appointments are often not made in the most appropriate clinic. Clinicians have lost control over organising their own clinics in a satisfactory way*

- *I am acute physician and do not therefore use C and B.*

- *Patients do not get to choose their doctor. All healthcare providers in a hospital or department are lumped together suggesting they all provide a similar service.*

60

- It works well for younger, computer literate patients, but not so well for elderly.

- We now have Unbook and Dictate - ie, the interception of bookings by administrators, even after they have been seen by a consultant and plans made, and pressure put on the patient to go to ….. TC. Talk about centralised, Stalinist medicine! What hypocrisy. They don't even inform the clinicians involved.

- Patients can only book where there are vacant appointment slots. the booking process is extremely complicated, telephone access often very limited and patients repeatedly tell of wrong appointments being sent out and multiple letters with different appointments being given

- Familiarity not equal to satisfaction or happiness

- We operate it using our secretarial staff. I do not believe it is time well spent in a consultation for a GP to be "on-line" searching for appointments.

- secretary helps out most of the time

- Not sure what is meant by online services.

- I'm an anaesthetist

- As a patient

- Generates excessive paper - all irrelevant front copies now filed in some hospitals. adds an unnecessary of layer of bureaucracy to a process which needs simplifying

- I don't know what you mean by online services - it the internet generally, or something more specific to C&B?

- Due to time constraints during consultation. I agreed with our secretary that she should refer anyone on Choose and Book who can be referred, and contact them to discuss the details. I have just been told that all those referrals last year don't count, as they have not been done by the doctor himself during the consultation (and I am already
- running late enough), and we do not get the payment for it. Sod Choose and Book!

- Familiar as a provider

- In general practice the slick use of online services during a consultation is normal; shame that the hospital computer system is so poor (I do know as I work in both locations!)

- Patients can't get through on the phone. They are told to ring back when appointments available, told they should not be booking their own appointments, advised not to use their choice but to accept a PCT preferred choice.

- I occasionally look at C&B and find it is no less horrible than the last time that I looked

- Nobody has ever specifically shown us how it works in real time, only the theory.

- As a consultant I am on the receiving end, so many of these statements do not apply to me

- I only see the end result at the hospital end.

- I am a hospital specialist so my contact with the system is now, mercifully, limited

- What a waste of money; typically not enough real (rather than enthusiast) GP input at the start, and dogmatic politics driving the service rather than need (it might satisfy a few patient wants instead)

- *As I say our secretaries do the searches etc. The doctors have the discussion with the patient about Provider choices.*
- *Too many incidents when c&b does not work and GP's are not informed of the problems. No technical support and little training.*

- *Adding letters too complicated.*

- *Slow and non-intuitive software*

- *Unreliable, not user friendly*

- *Wastes time and money*

- *The vast majority of our patients want to go to the local hospital, and many have got no transport to go anywhere else. Most of the foreign born patients don't understand anyway what they are supposed to do (poor command of English), and the elderly complain about "secret passwords and handshakes", they just want an appointment, at the local hospital, where they can get to on the bus.*

- *often difficult to find appropriate service. Time wasted trying to find unavailable services*

- *Poor functionality of system. patients are irritated by having booked appointments changed*

- *Poor selection of call back times for patients being fast track referred - patients are not always able to*
  Take calls at works and do not wish to tell colleagues that they have a possible cancer.

- *it often does not work especially at our branch surgery*

- *Like all web based services its fine when it works and disaster when it doesn't, so reliability is the Decisive factor*

- *We have no control over the Referral C+B managers' decisions to divert patients/alter appointments. It feels clinically very unsafe. It takes far too much of clinical consulting time up. Patients think we are mad to suggest they travel miles rather than use…….The ITCS are not on bus routes for patients without own transport but personal preference factors like this are ignored by C+B referral mangers. Despite numerous emails to ask for tech support not 1 has ever been answered or even acknowledged.*

- *Could have used "NA" as an option here... Not sure I've answered correctly*

- *Few GP's ever wanted it, my patients just want to go to the nearest hospital*

- *The main practical problem is that patient's appointments frequently get rescheduled. We try to persuade patients to take up appointments elsewhere - "choice" but most choose to be seen locally. The ability to book the appointment and know the timescale is helpful.*

- *What is the question here?*

- *poor patient experience - see above rigid if needs altering and very time consuming to try and alter appointments if necessary multiples paperwork and admin*

- *no experience*

- *Often we don't get to see referral letters until a few days before the appt, which means some could have been upgraded and some patients managed in a more efficient way*

- *What is the question?*

- *The wrong patients get to see the wrong doctors in the wrong time scale--creating a huge amount of unnecessary extra work*

- *PATIENTS NEEDING ENDOSOPCY ARE SENT TO CLINIC WHICH IS INAPPROPRIATE*

- *Reduces flexibility of booking and patients easily booked into inappropriate clinics maybe potential for better signposting*

- *What is the question?*

- *Requires additional time by member of the department to filter out referrals to wrong specialist*

- *We retrospectively check referrals to make sure patients are booked in the right clinic but still some have a wasted journey. The old system was much better, booking was done by the hospital and was more patient friendly*

- *Produces additional paperwork; yes the letters have to be photocopied for us to review! Adds pressure on over booked clinics and reduces time for complicated patients or those suffering complications.*

- *Excellent that we have a system that saves on-line copies of letters. Logos crash the system. Pts who change dates (for their own convenience) can then end up in wrong clinic. Attachments often don't come through.*

- *choose and book devalues choice; it is a cynical political idiom and devalues GP/ hospital consultant relationships. I would happily see it deconstructed and removed.*

- *I spend much of my time unpicking the mess C+B has made and rerouting patients to the appropriate place - and changing priority.*

- *No need for further comments. The system for booking appointments for our patients is MUCH WORSE than it was before. The patients don't like it, it doesn't work very well and it is very labour intensive, complex and expensive. In short, a disaster.*

- *We here in rural England have no true choice; it doesn't suit elderly patients*

- *From my perspective a referral letter still has to be dictated and typed. I agree patients experience may be improved if they have a desire to look beyond local delivery but few patients actually wish to.*

- *It actually increases the amount of work done by the patient*

- *Neutral means that I have no idea!*

- *Virtually no patients in our practice want to go anywhere other than …. and get worried if offered anywhere else*

- *Main benefit is that some patients with less complicated illnesses get seen more quickly*

- *In the past doctors could refer to any other doctor simply by writing a letter. You call CAB easier and simpler??*

- *Each referring consultation has a significant amt of time not talking about why the patient came in isn't this real job?? The secretary cd do this quicker & more effectively than I can !!!*

- *Patients want to be seen quickly and locally!!!*

- *Referrals out of area come with results from out of area. Continuity is important for many complex patients.*

- *Some patients eg elderly never action their referral as they find it too complicated.*

- *Patients even when offered choice usually want convenience - ie nearest Paperwork increases - lot of wasted paper giving sheets of instructions to patients Has no effect on unnecessary referrals More work fiddling with computer system during consultations - and more disgruntled patients as they are in consequence being "ignored"*

- *C+B definitely takes me more time than just dictating a letter*

- *the referral letters appear very confusing and cluttered*

- *Paper work is not reduced for GPS/Patients - it is increased.We now have an additional step in our referral process and numerous anxious patients unable to get through to the referral C+B number.*

- *We don't call it confuse and book for nothing.*

- *we are still getting inappropriate referrals - e.g.urology to paediatric medicine via C&B*

- *not so helpful when secondary care appointments arranged through chose and book are cancelled for no apparent reason and gps are asked to refer*

- *It is helpful to know that a referral has gone through and the system prevents GPs forgetting to write referral letters.*

- *No further comment required. It's a disaster.*

- *The main problem is medico-legal issues as above. The system has introduced unacceptable risk.*

- *Overall I think cob is a good idea and patients seem to like it and it gives them some power over their appt.*

- *Better education for doctors and patients about real benefits.*

- *The main problem is not on your list i.e. the process is too complex & should be simplified*

- *confidentiality issues continue - GPs often send full electronic patient history including sensitive social history*

- *I can adapt, change & don't mind learning new things, but C&B has made making referrals more difficult*

- *Scrap it!*

- *Main problem is lack of ability to refer to individual consultants by name. This prevents one person being responsible for the care of that patient.*

- *good local service would reduce need for choice*

- *have a simpler system practice secretaries cd deal with*

- *Disadvantages are lack of personal relationship of GP with hospital clinician. Less appropriate referral.*

- *Sort out the software and various interfaces - but is it really worth the cost*

- *These are all very value based questions!*

- The system should be patient centred rather than a data collection exercise

- Scrap the directory of services, probably the worst bit of the whole thing and re-implement from scratch. Streamline the whole thing.

- Additional personnel in clinics with overseeing consultant, rather than consultant seeing most patients.

- IF we had enough new pt gaps - would be better. We have GP's selecting new appt for 2 months time and then writing on the referral "urgent!"

- Scrap Choose & Book

- Uncouple OPD appointments from hospital and let private enterprises manage at and below tariff.

- Scrap it.

- PCT insists we use it.

- As such these changes are introduced - we make the best of them. They usually cost a lot of money and add very little to the real patient experience

- Take it way ASAP

- The system removes adequate clinical scrutiny in the process of referral which is detrimental to safe practice and therefore patient care. The process is viewed purely in administrative terms.

- there is no choice but to use it

- Do I have a choice?

- I will continue to use it as we are obliged to.

- given the choice I would prefer a different system

- Don't really have any choice, have to continue using it

- It will continue to be forced on us as providers I imagine--therefore no choice.

- I am not in any position to comment on the quality of care in hospitals far away, and we lost a lot of QOF points on the patient survey duet to doctors running late. If I have to do CAB during consultation myself, I shall run even later.
- Financially, there is no point continuing it, if the secretary is not allowed to do it. And if I had wanted to be a clerk, I should not have wasted my time at medical school.

- Likely to continue using as trust uses system Extra work generated as patients often put in wrong clinic and require additional admin to reappoint.
- Paper referrals still generated in order to screen them so no more efficient

- If we weren't paid to do it then I wouldn't

- We are required to use it

- I have no choice as a provider in continuing to use it. If I were the patient I would prefer not to use it.

- There are financial implications to us if we do not use the system. .

- We have no choice

- *we get paid for doing it so I will*

- *The genie is out of the bottle!*

- *The system has too many glitches, weaknesses that have had quick fix solutions and is now unwieldy, unworkable and requires each user to remember numerous idiosyncrasies for each service which may or may not appear that day. I would like a PCT manager to sit in on a busy GP surgery and observe the problems they have caused. Patient's complaints about the service are ignored.*

- *I'll have no say in whether we use it or not; it's a mode of referral in.*

- *(Satisfied isn't really the scale for likely to continue with it?)*

- *We don't have choice other than to use it*

- *I don't have any choice about whether its used for patients that I see - that decision is made by the trust/PCT*
- *Don't have any choice; it is a system forced into use by virtue of legal pressures and unhealthy inducements; wicked.*

- *Have to continue to use it - as a hospital consultant I have no choice!*

- *If I had the choice I would get rid of it*

- *Trust decision*

Conclusions

Recommendations

Action plan

Dear Colleague,

I am currently working with our Clinical Audit Department here at the ....Hospital, looking at the Choose and Book System. As a healthcare professional at the forefront of implementing this system, I would like to invite you to complete the following questionnaire in order to help us monitor how this service is being used and assess where improvements can be made. Your comments and thoughts are highly valued.

Your responses will be anonymously processed along with others. Every response will be treated with the strictest confidentially. You have the right to decline this invitation to participate. The results of this audit will be disseminated through a report that will be published through the Audit Department.

Your participation in completing this online questionnaire is most appreciated, it takes approximately 5 minutes to complete. Try and complete the survey on one sitting. Thank you for taking the time to complete this questionnaire which can be accessed simply by clicking on the link given below. Could you kindly complete it as soon as possible?

http://www.surveymonkey.com/s/YNPJ6PB

References –
1. http://www.chooseandbook.nhs.uk/
2   http://www.surveymonkey.com

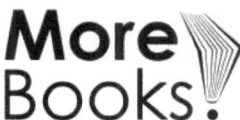
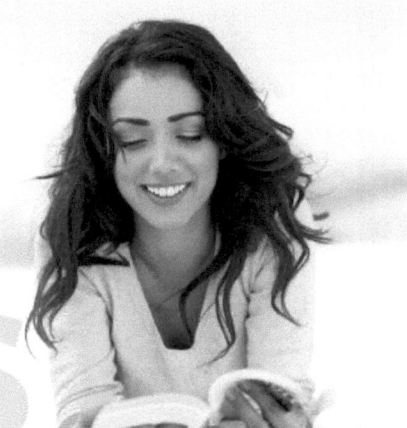

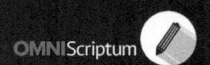

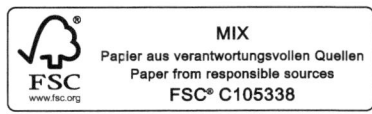
Printed by Books on Demand GmbH, Norderstedt / Germany